Ride the Tiger
to the Mountain

A PORTABLE STANFORD BOOK

Ride the Tiger to the Mountain

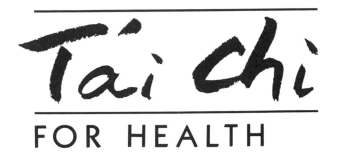

FOR HEALTH

Martin and Emily Lee
and JoAn Johnstone

Addison-Wesley Publishing Company, Inc.
Reading, Massachusetts   Menlo Park, California   New York
Don Mills, Ontario   Wokingham, England   Amsterdam
Bonn   Sydney   Singapore   Tokyo   Madrid   San Juan

This edition is published by arrangement with the Stanford Alumni Association.

This book is not intended, nor should it be regarded, as medical advice. For such advice you should consult your doctor. Neither the publisher nor the authors may be held responsible for any damage, direct or indirect, that may be caused or exacerbated by activities described in this book.

Library of Congress Cataloging-in-Publication Data

Lee, Martin, 1936–
    Ride the tiger to the mountain: t'ai chi for health/by Martin Lee, Emily Lee, and JoAn Johnstone.
        p.   cm.   —(A Portable Stanford book)
    ISBN 0-201-18077-4
    1. T'ai chi ch'üan.   I. Lee, Emily.   II. Johnstone, JoAn.
III. Title.
GV504.L43, 1989
613.7'148—dc20   89-6622
                                                                 CIP

Book and cover design by Andrea Hendrick
Photography by Lynn Hunton
Drawings by Sylvia MacBride
Set in 11-point Palatino by Terry Robinson & Co., Inc., San Francisco, CA

ABCDEFGHIJ-HA-89
First printing, April 1989

This book is dedicated with respect and gratitude
to our mentors Master Kuo Lien-Yin and
Professor Yu Pen-Shi, M.D.

CONTENTS

ACKNOWLEDGMENTS

We are grateful for the assistance of many people who participated at various stages in the production of this book. Della van Heyst provided us with valuable guidance and spiritual support since our idea of writing this book was first conceived five years ago. JoAn Johnstone, our co-author, has done a superb job of describing our ideas and experience in her beautiful and accurate English. She has also made a major contribution to the organization of the material.

We would also like to thank the team who helped us with the production of the book: Miriam Miller for her editing; Gayle Hemenway for her skill in design and production; Sylvia MacBride for her excellent illustrations; Andrea Hendrick for her cover and book design; Lynn Hunton for his photographs; and Herbert Weidner for his editorial comments.

Many of our friends and colleagues helped in our study of Ch'i with Professor Yu: Professor Willard Fee, Professor Thomas Finger, Professor Herbert Benson, Professor Craig Heller, and Professor Ralph Burger. We are especially grateful to our godmother Ou-Yang Min for her participation in our study.

The response of many of our students has been of great value. They have been our source of encouragement and inspiration, especially in the personal experiences we are sharing with you in this book.

Our children Joyce and Bryce have been helpful in organizing and proofreading the many versions of the manuscript, and Melinda for contributing special ideas. Finally, we thank Professor Chuang Yin for the lovely calligraphy and Professor Archie Bahm for his enlightening thoughts.

A T'ai Chi Fable

A T'ai Chi master came to the village to catch a
   tiger.
Upon finding the tiger, the master looked into
   the tiger's eyes.
Without any struggle, the tiger fell to its knees.
The Master sat on the tiger's back and rode the
   tiger to the mountain.

The Moral: Anyone could master oneself by
   looking inward.

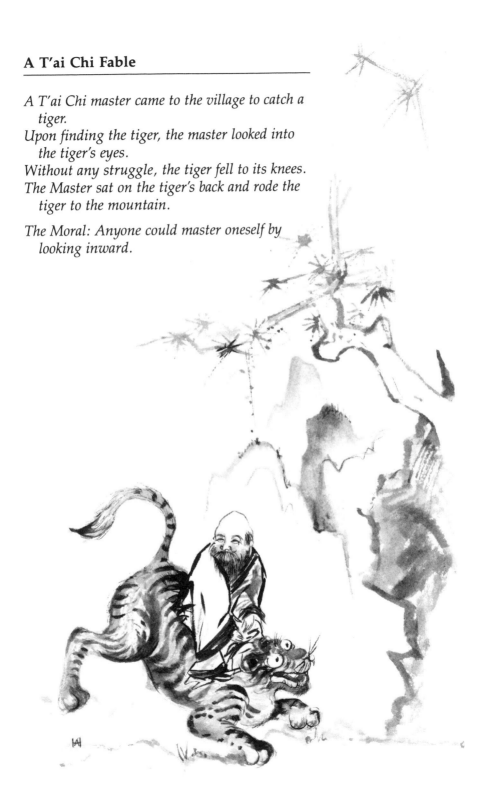

INTRODUCTION

We live in an age of science, an age of technological innovation. Though the population of the United States is aging, this aging has occurred, in part, because new knowledge and new techniques in medicine, science, and technology have helped to extend human life. We live not only in an unusual time but in a special place. Ours is a country marked by a rare cultural diversity. These facts are so familiar that we may forget how remarkable they are and how unique is this time and place in which we live.

The connections between these facts are also remarkable. Although in many times and places cultural diversity has led to endless destructive conflict, this country as a whole—and states like California in particular—have been enriched by a diversity that includes not only races and nationalities but also ideas. In recent decades even scientific disciplines have benefited from the melting pot. One result of this mingling and diversity has been an outpouring of scientific knowledge from which we receive many benefits every day. Our country and our state lead the world in cultural diversity and in new knowledge.

This is a state of affairs we should enjoy. Fortunately, many Americans, including some of the most thoughtful among us, are learning to reap personal benefits from scientific knowledge and cultural diversity by pursuing *internal* knowledge—personal knowledge of the world of body and mind within us. By means as new and technical as biofeedback and as ancient and inward as yoga and T'ai Chi, they are finding ways to reduce stress, preserve youth, and enhance good health. During the past decade, more and more people have begun to practice a range of disciplines learned from India, Tibet, Japan, and China, disciplines that teach them, and train them, to look inside themselves. These disciplines teach "internal practices"—meditation, yoga, and martial arts—and centers for the study of such practices have opened in every major city. Many of these disciplines share a common goal—to help us stay younger and become healthier inside and out.

Historically, China has been the melting pot of many of these internal practices. Long ago, the Chinese combined practices originating in India with their own disciplines in philosophy, medicine, and martial arts. Breathing exercises, Ch'i Kung (pronounced "chee gung"), and meditations were practiced for centuries in many well-known monasteries and schools of martial arts. In some monasteries, the monks practiced martial arts. In some schools of martial arts, the students practiced meditation. In China, self-defense and philosophy have long been integrated into a single discipline.

Wall rubbings found in China and dated as far back as 3000 years ago illustrate the process of healing exercises. These exercises, which were generally stationary, focused a person's attention on breathing, in order to send energy throughout the body. They developed into the system of Ch'i Kung, which uses breathing both to direct the amount of *ch'i*, that is, energy, flowing through the body and to keep the flow itself unobstructed. Within the martial arts, which took form after these healing exercises had been developed, a branch called "internal martial arts" evolved. These exercises integrated Ch'i Kung exercises with martial arts movements to develop the power of ch'i for self-defense. T'ai Chi (pronounced "tie-jee"), as one of the internal martial arts, incorporates Ch'i Kung, as well as meditation and physical movements.

In this book, we have chosen to concentrate on the Ch'i Kung and meditation aspects of T'ai Chi—the self-healing rather than the self-defense aspects. By doing the exercises, you relax your body, get your ch'i flowing, and free your thoughts. The benefits should come quickly: release of stress, more energy, and freedom from psychosomatic illness.

Because I grew up in China, I had the privilege of being exposed to and influenced by this great heritage. After coming to the United States, I was educated in engineering and physics and worked in the field of automated process control and system optimization. For more than thirty years I have worked in the fields of science and engineering. For more than twenty years I have practiced and studied the martial arts, Ch'i Kung, and meditation, becoming a T'ai Chi master and teacher. I myself have become a melting pot of scientific knowledge and diverse cultural traditions. Now I am able to combine my scientific methods with ancient traditions not only to practice and teach T'ai Chi but also to understand how and why it works. Through this book I would like to share with you my T'ai Chi and Ch'i Kung practices.

For me, youth is the central fact of my experience with T'ai Chi and Ch'i Kung: the practice of these internal exercises has given me knowledge of how to stay younger. My study has brought me health, peace, and wisdom as well. But the gift that most surprised me— and the gift that seems a daily miracle—is a youthful vitality of body and mind that seems never to diminish. Youthfulness was the first quality that drew me to my teachers, who were far from young. Now it is a quality that I find in myself and that, through this book, I hope to share with you.

I am fortunate to have studied T'ai Chi, Ch'i Kung, and meditation with two great masters from China. For more than ten years, I studied T'ai Chi in San Francisco with Master Kuo Lien-Ying, the fourth grand master in the Yang family T'ai Chi martial arts system descended from Yang's elder son. (The second grand master, Yang Pan-Hou, was T'ai Chi teacher to the emperor in the final years of the Ch'ing dynasty, which ended in 1912.) For more than two years, I had a live-in Ch'i Kung master, Professor Yu Pen-Shi, M.D., a grand master of the Hsing Yi martial arts system and a Tibetan Buddhist teacher. My wife, Emily, and I were trained intensively in Ch'i Kung by Professor Yu. In the Chinese martial arts tradition, it is a great honor to be accepted as a disciple or a godson—in my case, as a disciple of Master Kuo and a godson of Professor Yu. For more than six years I have been studying Ch'i Kung, or healing exercises, with my godmother, Ou-Yang Ming, who, at the age of eighty, was chosen best woman martial arts teacher of 1987 by *Inside Kung Fu*, a magazine of the martial arts. Emily and I are founders of the T'ai Chi Cultural Center, an organization for study and research into T'ai Chi for healing, health, harmony, and happiness. We have been teaching T'ai Chi the Ch'i Kung way for more than fifteen years.

During the writing of this book I realized that the technical and the nontechnical work I do is the same. My technical work is finding a way to optimize the performance of an accelerator, a device for moving charged particles (electrons) at high velocities. My nontechnical work is finding a way to optimize my own performance. The method is the same in both cases. The only difference is the application of the method: in one case the application is external, in the other it is internal.

Let me explain what I mean by drawing a comparison from my technical world. As an engineer, I have always believed that how well an accelerator operates depends on how it is controlled. About fifteen years ago, as a physicist, I introduced the concept of the model-based control system in order to improve the operation of the accelerators at Stanford. This model-based control method is known as a "top-down" method, in contrast to the conventional "bottom-up" method. In a top-down control system, the performance of an accelerator depends on the model. The more intelligence we can put into the model, the better the accelerator performs. In order to make the model more intelligent, I have applied the most sophisticated techniques used in the field of artificial intelligence to find ways to improve the model. (This process creates what is called an "expert system.") Because of the success we have achieved at the Stanford Linear Accelerator Center (SLAC), every modern accelerator around the world is controlled by this technique.

The connection between the performance of an accelerator and its control system revealed to me a similar connection between personal well-being and self-control. My experience suggested that the same top-down method that makes an accelerator run efficiently can be used to improve self-control. What I am introducing in this book is a mind-based control system for improving self-control.

To a physicist, nature is uniform as well as complex. The same materials and the same forces are to be observed in the operation of particle accelerators and in the life processes of human beings. Once I had seen this analogy between the model that controls an accelerator and the internal practices that control the human mind, I was not surprised that some of the oldest physical disciplines in the world— T'ai Chi Ch'uan, Ch'i Kung, and meditation—should draw upon the same principles that could produce an innovation in the art of accelerator control.

In a top-down control system for human beings, well-being begins with the mind. The more intelligent the mind, the more the potential for well-being. In order to make my mind more intelligent, I have practiced the sophisticated techniques used in meditation and the martial arts—principally T'ai Chi Ch'uan—to find ways to improve my own mind. After twenty years of practicing T'ai Chi, I feel as young as ever, both physically and mentally. Because of my personal experience and success, I have been able to teach and demonstrate these sophisticated internal practices to many students. Emily and I have found that all of our students are enjoying similar benefits with varying degrees of success. Some of their stories and comments are included as illustrations of the power of T'ai Chi.

Many of our students have suffered from asthma, arthritis, headaches, high blood pressure, and backaches. Their success in healing these illnesses or in keeping them under control has been among the most remarkable effects of their learning. My own total recovery from allergies and asthma, from which I suffered for fifteen years before practicing T'ai Chi Ch'uan, is a personal success story. My students have experienced recoveries just as spectacular. One of these students is a seventy-year-old who had suffered arthritis in her fingers, hips, and shoulders for more than twenty years. Now she is able to play golf and teach tap dancing. She has recently had a face-lift so that she could have "a face to match her body." In this book, I would like to provide some insight into how such healing works and to introduce the Ch'i Kung techniques that promote it through the practice of T'ai Chi Ch'uan.

T'ai Chi Ch'uan is an internal martial art, internal because it is based on working inside one's system, inside of the mind and body. Inside the mind, it works on the control of our thoughts. Inside the body, it works on the control of our energy or ch'i. Since T'ai Chi is also a top-down method that connects mind (top) to body (bottom), it thus works on the mind, body, thoughts, and ch'i simultaneously. This combination makes T'ai Chi the most effective way of gaining self-control. The different rates of success for each student depend on how diligently he or she practices T'ai Chi, following the techniques described in the instructional part of this book.

It is impossible to learn T'ai Chi by simply reading the book. This is internal learning, and you must practice the exercises in order to learn. Reading and practicing go hand in hand. Reading the material will also help your practice. Soon you will learn how to think and what to feel as you practice the movements.

Learning T'ai Chi is a slow process. The twelve movements described in the book typically take our students three months to learn. Take your time. Don't rush through them. Learn one new step and practice it for a week before learning the next one. Always remember to use your mind and not just your body.

I would like to pay tribute to my teachers. Master Kuo was in his seventies and Professor Yu in his eighties when Emily and I studied with them. (Master Kuo started to learn from his teacher when that master was more than 100 years old.) They were ageless. They were younger and more intelligent than I was. They were living symbols of how we can be young at any age. With twenty more years of practice, I am looking forward to being as young as they.

Martin Lee
Los Altos, California
August, 1988

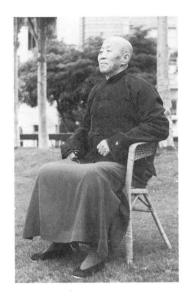 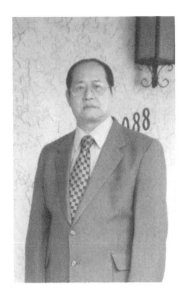

Master Kuo Lien-Ying   **Professor Yu Pen-Shi, M.D.**

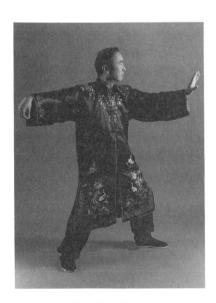

Martin Lee

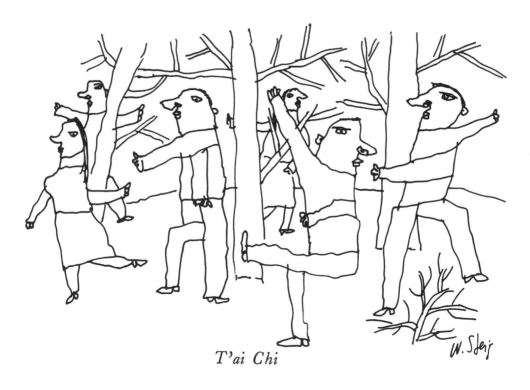

T'ai Chi

A NEW APPROACH TO T'AI CHI CH'UAN

WHAT IS T'AI CHI CH'UAN?

Think of a time when you felt at ease—tranquil, at peace, and filled with a sense of well-being. All of us know moments like these, times when we are happy, radiant with health, and buoyant with a sense of steady inner strength. For most of us, though, such moments of fullness and ease, calm and confidence, come rarely, the lucky accidents of a happy day. Most of us, too, can recall that when we were younger, we more often felt such a spontaneous sense of well-being.

What, then, if someone taught you how to create feelings like these every day and to prolong and intensify them? What if you could capture, every day, a sensation of moving fluidly, effortlessly, at will, with mind and body working in unison? What if you could carry a sense of well-being into every day, a cushion against unpleasantness and stress? And what if this sense of well-being came for free and brought with it only other good effects—would you not feel that someone had given you a great treasure? That is what you will feel when you learn T'ai Chi Ch'uan.

T'AI CHI GIVES MORE THAN YOU EXPECT

In the nearly twenty years that we have taught T'ai Chi we have seen how T'ai Chi surprises almost every student. After the first few weeks of study, students experience a new relaxation, power of concentration, and flow of energy. In our classes, students' ages generally range over six decades, yet the same benefits come to all students, whatever their age. But let them speak for themselves.[1]

A technical editor:
I have much more energy since learning T'ai Chi. People are always surprised to learn my age. At 40, I'm more active and vigorous than ever. I continually take on new challenges, but it gets easier rather than harder. I have greater confidence and concentration and am stronger than ever before.

A teacher:
I hoped for more self-confidence because T'ai Chi is a martial art, but I never expected T'ai Chi to improve my ability to concentrate. Sometimes now my ability to focus is so intense it's scary. I think twice sometimes about reading something because I know I'll get into it so deeply. I think, "Do I really want to learn all that?"

A pianist:
I always thought you had to tense your muscles to express energy and force. Now I understand that you can make a movement full of energy and power that is completely relaxed.

A computer scientist:
T'ai Chi contributes great inner peace and balance to everything I do, however big or small. It pervades my existence—without my trying. It has enabled me to integrate all aspects of my life and to attain a detachment that minimizes the effects of otherwise stressful situations. My mental and physical abilities have increased by leaps and bounds. As the focus of a way of life, it reinforces a positive attitude, a sensible and moderate diet, a healthful environment, and close personal ties; it has become a source of continual rejuvenation for me.

And a professor:
When I do T'ai Chi, I feel I start every day with an advantage.

These are the feelings—the inner strengths—that daily practice of T'ai Chi creates. When I began to study T'ai Chi seriously, I was in my early thirties. My motive was simple: I was in poor health. I hoped these exercises would help me to heal my body and to regain my strength. To encourage me in what would be an arduous project, my wife, Emily, joined with me. Thanks to T'ai Chi, I regained not only strength but full health, happiness, and a sense of well-being I had not known for many years. We learned a set of exercises one step at a time; performing them daily transformed and renewed our lives. Thus, when we began to teach T'ai Chi, our motive was gratitude to our teacher, Master Kuo, who had placed this great gift in our hands.

A SET OF SLOW MOVEMENTS

T'ai Chi Ch'uan (pronounced "tie-jee choowan") is a set of slow, continuous, evenly paced and carefully patterned natural movements based upon the principle of shifting one's weight while keeping the body stable and upright. The movements are connected by smooth, even breathing. They are characterized by circularity of motion and relaxation of tension. Each movement begins in the mind and is directed by a conscious mental intention.

In T'ai Chi, the mind has a double role. It is the source of *intention*, directing and controlling movement, and *attention*, monitoring the effects of movement. Someone watching T'ai Chi sees only the slowness and the beauty of the movements. Someone doing T'ai Chi is wholly involved in guiding a stream of energy and enjoying an experience of attentive awareness.

A SPECIAL APPROACH TO T'AI CHI

Many people think of T'ai Chi Ch'uan as a martial art. They are correct; it is a powerful martial art. Yet T'ai Chi is much more. It is also an art of the mind and a health-giving art. For this reason, our approach to T'ai Chi is not through the martial arts but through those fundamental aspects of T'ai Chi that give it its power. Our aim is to introduce students to the essence of T'ai Chi.

In its essence, T'ai Chi has a close relationship with another, even more ancient art, the healing art of Ch'i Kung. It is through Ch'i Kung that we approach T'ai Chi. Each art has its special strength.

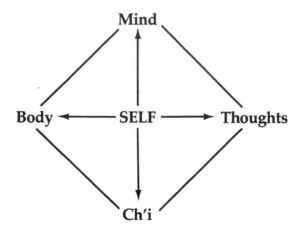

Figure 1-1
This figure shows schematically how T'ai Chi develops self-control. T'ai Chi movements begin as an intention in the mind; they are guided by thoughts. The body's energy, or ch'i, responds to mental intentions. The body, too, follows mental directions. By the practice of controlling these components of action, the self strengthens its power over mind and body. This strengthening we call self-control.

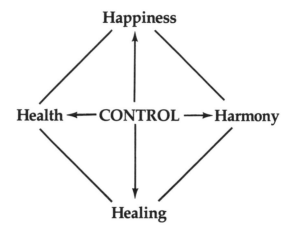

Figure 1-2
This figure shows how an improvement in self-control can enhance your whole life. The self we seek through T'ai Chi has the power to heal its injuries, and thus achieve health. It possesses a quiet inner happiness, and lives in harmony with others. Each of these powers—for healing, health, happiness, and harmony—depends upon the others. For example, the happier we feel the better we get along with others, while the more harmonious our social lives the less tension we feel and the better our health and the greater our powers of recovery (healing). Self-control stands at the center of a synergistic system.

Ch'i Kung (pronounced "chee gung") is the practice of controlling the flow of energy—ch'i—within the body through breathing and mental intention. Most Ch'i Kung exercises are stationary, although some use circular rotations to stimulate the flow of energy. They emphasize relaxation and breathing evenly. Approaching T'ai Chi through Ch'i Kung allows students to experience the essential nature of T'ai Chi more fully and more rapidly than by other methods.

These two arts complement each other. Simply put, both T'ai Chi and Ch'i Kung do four essential things: strengthen the link between mind and body, improve self-control (in every sense, from control over physical movement to control over emotions), relax and calm both mind and body, and promote healing and rejuvenation.

We approach T'ai Chi as an art that promotes the wholeness of the self through self-control. Because T'ai Chi movements begin as a mental intention and are guided by thought, T'ai Chi improves self-control by linking mind and body. This linking is a firm and close one because the flow of energy in the body (ch'i) is sensitive to mental direction. With practice, one can bring mind, thoughts, ch'i, and body into a harmony under one's control. (See Figure 1-1.)

ABOUT THIS BOOK

By following the instructions in this book, a student should be able to learn T'ai Chi in three to six months with daily practice of ten to twenty minutes. In three to four months, you will become familiar with twelve T'ai Chi movements and six healing Ch'i Kung exercises. Within this time, with daily practice, you should begin to feel the essential benefits of T'ai Chi. (See Figure 1-2.)

In our course, students make the most dramatic gains in the early weeks, the period when they learn these twelve movements, the first of a full series of sixty-four. It is with these fundamental movements that we introduce students to T'ai Chi.

The illustrated manual will guide you step-by-step through the movements and exercises. Through this manual you will discover how accessible T'ai Chi really is: it takes no equipment, it causes no sore muscles, it takes little time. You will also find that T'ai Chi is practical. You can use it for many purposes: to relax and become more calm, to develop better coordination for tennis or stronger legs for skiing, to build confidence, to keep flexible, and even to age without feeling older. You should not be surprised if, whatever you seek, you find more.

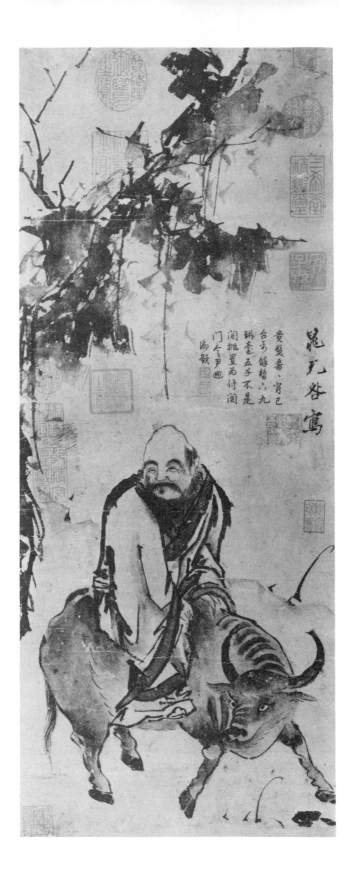

NATURE, ENERGY, AND T'AI CHI

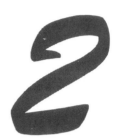

Nature is great because it is simple.
Lao Tzu, *Tao Teh King*[1]

I sing the body electric!
Walt Whitman

The soul is not more than the body,
And the body
is not more than the soul
And there is no object so soft but it makes a hub
*   for the wheel'd universe.*
Walt Whitman, *Song of Myself*

Nature and Nature's laws lay hid in night:
God said "Let Newton be!" and all was light.
Alexander Pope

When Newton declared that one force pulls an apple to earth and planets toward the sun, he revealed to his contemporaries the deepest secrets of nature. A mathematical genius, Newton stated the laws of motion, explaining the universe as a machine, something like a well-designed clock.

Because these laws seemed to prove that the universe works like a machine, it confirmed a similar view of human beings. Years before Newton's discovery, Descartes had pictured the human being as a spirit living in a material body, something like a pilot in an airplane. In his view, mind and body shared almost nothing, because they were made of different stuff. When Descartes imagined a connection between mind and body, he pictured a kind of on/off switch in the center of the brain, located in a pinecone-shaped structure called the pineal gland. Through this center, he believed, a thinking mind animated a mechanical body.

As to the human conditions of sickness and health, they belonged only to the body: "My thought," Descartes said, "compares a sick man and an ill-made clock with my idea of a healthy man and a well-made clock."[2] A person's feelings, thoughts, and attitudes could have no influence on the body, just as a clockmaker's thoughts about a clock would have no effect on how well it ran.

Although we no longer believe the universe runs like a clock, the seventeenth-century view of mind and body still has some influence on our thinking. The brain is often described as a kind of machine—the computer is now the favorite comparison—and the mind a separate spiritual entity somehow attached to it. Many psychotherapists still do not greatly concern themselves with the condition of a patient's body, and many physicians still do not ask patients about their feelings and thoughts.

AN EASTERN VIEW OF NATURE

In contrast, the Eastern understanding of nature emphasizes unity rather than division between mind and body. Furthermore, describing how mind and body function, the Eastern view emphasizes patterns of flow rather than regular mechanisms.

In *The Wandering Taoist*, Deng Ming Dao tells a Chinese creation myth. In the beginning, according to the myth, only pure life energy, or ch'i, existed. This energy gave rise to everything that now exists:

the dynamic balance of emptiness and fullness (*yin* and *yang*), the perfect intermingling of emptiness and fullness (*T'ai Chi*), the five elements (water, metal, wood, fire, and earth), and human beings. The universe remains in flux, oscillating between poles of emptiness (yin) and fullness (yang).

The myth also tells how human beings fell from the perfection of their original state. Created as microcosms of the universe, humans contained the elements in a changing cycle and the oscillating balance of yin and yang. Most important, the life energy, or ch'i, flowed unhindered through them just as it flowed through the universe. Thus created, humans had prodigious powers. They had great strength, they could fly, and they could understand themselves and the universe.

But the human race abused its power. Therefore the gods decided to hobble the created upstarts. This they did by limiting the flow of life energy in and through each human being. To block the flow of ch'i, three gates were placed along the human spine: one at the tailbone, one at the shoulder blades, and one at the base of the skull. Thus checked, humans lost their extravagant powers.[3]

The traditional goal of T'ai Chi then became reestablishment of the original unfettered connection between the life energy in the universe and the life energy in each human being. Equally, the exercises of T'ai Chi Ch'uan helped humans to reconstruct within themselves the equilibrium of T'ai Chi, a physical state in which yin and yang, emptiness and fullness, perfectly intermingle.

THE MEANING OF THE WORD CH'I

The Chinese character for ch'i has two parts: The upper is the character for "air," the lower is the character for "rice."

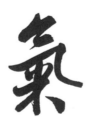

The word *ch'i* has more than two hundred uses. For example, "sky ch'i" is weather, "lightning ch'i" is electrical power, "brewing ch'i" means getting angry, and "money ch'i" means getting rich.

In medicine and the martial arts, ch'i means life energy. From the human perspective, ch'i is the energy in the air we breathe and in the food we eat. The body converts air and food to energy, and it distributes this energy to every cell in the body. Because the health of the body depends upon the health of each cell in the body, optimal health depends upon a full and continuous flow of ch'i.

Whether ch'i is to be treated as a concept or a fact can be a puzzle. Fritjof Capra, author of *The Tao of Physics*, explains ch'i in this way:

> The word literally means "gas" or "ether" and was used in ancient China to denote the vital breath or energy animating the cosmos. But neither of these Western terms describes the concept adequately. *Ch'i* is not a substance, nor does it have the purely quantitative meaning of our scientific concept of energy. It is used in Chinese medicine in a very subtle way to describe the various patterns of flow and fluctuation in the human organism, as well as the continual exchanges between organism and environment. *Ch'i* does not refer to the flow of any particular substance but rather seems to represent the principle of flow as such, which, in the Chinese view, is always cyclical.[4]

On the other hand, David Eisenberg, a medical exchange student from Harvard University studying at the Institute of Traditional Chinese Medicine in Beijing, was told firmly by a senior member of the faculty that ch'i is a fact:

> You are the first American medical exchange student to study traditional medicine in the People's Republic of China. If you are to accomplish your objective, then you must be convinced of the existence of Ch'i. Without Ch'i there is no Chinese medicine. Without an understanding of Ch'i, Western medicine, with all its powerful science, will remain ignorant of the single greatest gift of Chinese medicine. It is real, this Ch'i, and you should make every effort while you are in China to study it—to be convinced of its significance.[5]

Another of Eisenberg's teachers, a professor of anatomy, explained that ch'i ("that which differentiates life from death, animate from inanimate")[6] is inherited in finite quantity from one's parents. It is augmented and replenished by ch'i extracted from food and air. It flows through the body through specific channels and flows through every organ.

Ill health develops when the flow of ch'i becomes stagnant or imbalanced. The aim of traditional medicine is to regulate the flow of ch'i through acupuncture, acupressure massage (massage focused on sensitive pressure points), and herbal remedies. By these means, Eisenberg was told, the body's equilibrium is restored:

> All of human pathology can be seen in terms of balances and imbalances. A balanced state corresponds to health. Any excess or deficiency corresponds to illness. When the body is in a state of equilibrium, internally and with respect to the external environment, then it possesses a "positive vitality," a form of Ch'i that protects the body and defends it from "pathogenic factors."[7]

In Western terms, a balanced flow of ch'i enhances the ability of the body's immune system to resist disease.

At the Xiyuan hospital in Beijing, researchers now study Ch'i Kung, and the doctors who can do so treat patients by Ch'i Kung techniques. In such cases the doctor works directly with the patient's ch'i, using his own ch'i the way an acupuncturist uses a needle. One of the few practitioners of this skill, Dr. Yang Bao-Tang, explained to a reporter for the *New York Times* in 1986, "Through Ch'i Kung, a powerful force, my 'Ch'i' comes from my hand, and the patient will feel it inside his body. The 'Ch'i' moves from my body and has a physical effect on the patient."[8]

The reporter watched Dr. Yang on a home visit working with a paralyzed woman. He moved his hands rhythmically through the air, palms toward the patient, until the patient responded, her arms and body echoing his movements. With Dr. Yang's help, the young woman lifted her hands above her head and moved her body from side to side. He exercised her muscles in this way for about half an hour.

The patient explained that she felt the ch'i as "a kind of force that tries to lift my arms. Sometimes it's a bit warm. I feel something in my arms. I can make my arms move. I can feel something in my body." The patient's father, a scientist, said he believed that the treatments had helped to improve his daughter's condition but that he could not understand how or why, given the framework of scientific inquiry he was accustomed to use. "I don't know what it is," he said. "If I was forced to say what it might be, I suppose I would say maybe it is an electromagnetic phenomenon. But I really don't know." This theory receives support from the fact that acupuncture pressure points, points at which ch'i is more easily touched and controlled, "have distinct electrical resistance and thermosensitivity, unlike other areas at the body surface."[9]

FURTHER SUPPORT FOR THE ELECTRICAL THEORY

The extraordinary abilities of Li Qing-Hong also lend support to the theory that Ch'i Kung is manipulation of the body's electrical system. Li Qing-Hong, who is 35, began to practice Ch'i Kung when he was 15; he treats patients by projecting ch'i and by transmitting an electrical current to them. Like Dr. Yang, Li can exercise paralytic patients by moving their arms and legs with the force of his own energy. A reporter who observed one of Li's sessions watched as a patient, a 58-year-old man partially paralyzed by a stroke, moved his arms and legs, mirroring the movements of Li, who stood behind him. But Li has another ability as well, one which he discovered by accident when he noticed that he could alter the volume of his transistor radio at will without touching it.

Li began to practice controlling electricity. He now treats patients at the Railway Ministry Hospital on the western outskirts of Beijing by touching them with live electric wires (220 volts) that he holds in his hands. Touching the reporter on the palm with a wire, he said, "You would be electrocuted if you tried to touch these wires on your own. I am controlling the current."[10] The reporter's thumb twitched, and the current felt "warm, ticklish." Li then demonstrated the power of the current flowing through his hands by spearing "a piece of frozen fish with two copper spits, each connected to a wire from a wall outlet." Nothing happened. Li then took a spit in each hand and, according to the reporter, "Smoke begins to curl up from the fish, which starts to hiss and crackle." The current, said Li, was passing through his hands and cooking the fish. He asked the reporter to feel his fingertips. They were cool.

Though claims that electrical current has curative powers are generally viewed with skepticism by doctors, a researcher at the University of Southern California has found "a promising non-surgical way to treat life-threatening bleeding ulcers by coagulating the blood with electrical current."[11]

A HSING YI AND CH'I KUNG MASTER

Our teacher, Dr. Yu Pen-Shi, was a Hsing Yi martial arts master and also a renowned Ch'i Kung master. Dr. Yu, who had attended a German-Chinese high school in Hankow, Hupeh, was also Western trained. By a stroke of luck he received his medical degree in Germany. When he was studying medicine in Shanghai, a ship of the Hamburg-American line came to the medical college hospital looking for a German-speaking doctor to replace the ship's doctor. After the young Yu sailed with the ship to Germany, the company supported him in Heidelberg, where he earned an M.D. in gynecology and dermatology. Returning to Shanghai in 1927, he became a professor concurrently at Tung Teh Medical College and Southeast Medical College. From 1949 until his retirement in 1966, he was chief of the department of dermatology at the Shanghai First People's Hospital and was recognized as one of China's eminent dermatologists.

On returning to China from Germany, Dr. Yu began to study Shiao-Lin boxing, a tough, aggressive martial art from which karate is derived, and Hsing Yi, an internal martial art more like T'ai Chi, in which intelligent use of strength overcomes force.[12] (Hsing Yi is named for "hsing," or "physical form," and "yi," or "mental intention.") Some historians believe that Hsing Yi martial art can be traced as far back as the Southern Sung Dynasty (1127–1379).

Dr. Yu's Hsing Yi teacher was Wang Xiang-Zhai, who trained his Hsing Yi students in the healing exercises of Ch'i Kung and who was the first grand master to do so publicly. Wang was successor to Kuo Yuen-Shin (no relation to my Master Kuo), a turn-of-the-century contemporary of Yang Pan-Hou and a grand master of equal fame, of whom it was said, "With one hand he could punch his way across China." Among his skills, Kuo had the ability to project ch'i. Dr. Yu hoped to learn the skill from Wang.

Accordingly, Dr. Yu studied Ch'i Kung with Wang for five years, giving him gifts, even a house to live in and servants to staff it. Unfortunately, Wang lacked knowledge of how to project ch'i. Kuo had one day promised to teach the skill to Wang, but the old master had died without sharing his technique. Nonetheless, Dr. Yu's technique in Hsing Yi grew so powerful that he succeeded his teacher as the grand master of the Hsing Yi martial arts system. He also continued to work diligently to develop the ability to project ch'i. With the help of a T'ai Chi master, he at last found that he could do so. Combining this rare skill with his technique in Hsing Yi, he became famous as a martial arts master who could repel opponents without touching them—simply by the projection of his ch'i.

Our T'ai Chi teacher in San Francisco, Master Kuo Lien-Ying, like Dr. Yu, had studied Hsing Yi with Wang Xiang-Zhai. In this way, he had learned of Dr. Yu's remarkable skill. Fascinated by the phenomenon of ch'i projection, I determined to bring Dr. Yu to the United States through a university program for visiting scholars.

To discover the whereabouts of Dr. Yu, however, was not easy, for China was then filled with the turmoil of the Cultural Revolution, which disrupted normal life and, among other things, shut down all medical schools between 1966 and 1971. During the Cultural Revolution, a man like Dr. Yu was doubly in danger, as a Western-trained physician and, equally, as a practitioner of traditional arts like Hsing Yi and Ch'i Kung. Indeed, as I learned later, Dr. Yu had spent two years of the Cultural Revolution confined to a room, though not formally imprisoned.

At last, with the help of a professor at the Stanford School of Medicine (and with help, too, from Dr. Herbert Benson of the Harvard Medical School), I was able to bring Dr. Yu to Palo Alto in 1980. As a visiting scholar, he would take part in studies of ch'i. These studies, at Stanford and at the University of California at Santa Cruz, showed that Dr. Yu, like many who have long practiced meditation, had the ability to lower his heart rate and breathing rate and to change the pattern of alpha waves in his brain. He also possessed an ability that the researchers found very unusual, the ability to reduce the movement of his eyes to an undetectable level during meditation.

Although the studies with Dr. Yu measured the effect of ch'i, they failed to measure ch'i itself. Several experiments, however, did turn up some facts of interest about the phenomenon of projection of ch'i.[13] Like the paralytic patients described earlier, subjects separated from Dr. Yu by a one-way glass moved in response to ch'i. On the other hand, a copper barrier seemed to reduce the transmission of ch'i. A complicating factor, though, was this: the recipient's training was also a factor in reception. This discovery was not altogether surprising. In acupuncture, the doctor must "catch" the ch'i of a patient by twirling a needle, and the patient must cooperate, telling the doctor when he has caught the ch'i. Similarly, in these experiments, the transmission was stronger if the receiver had already learned to be sensitive to the flow of ch'i.

A PERSONAL EXPERIENCE OF CH'I PROJECTION

While Dr. Yu was a visiting professor, Emily and I practiced meditation, martial arts exercises, and Ch'i Kung with him daily. He and his wife were our houseguests. We learned that he could indeed project his ch'i and even, as an expression of his mental intention, control its intensity. After we had been practicing with him for about a year, we could feel the projected energy to varying degrees, ranging from a gentle repellent force to a powerful one like a jolt from an electric wire.

My first experience of Dr. Yu's power to project ch'i was unforgettable. We were conducting an experiment in the study of ch'i, and we had gathered a group of students of the martial arts, for Dr. Yu was teaching Ch'i Kung to many of the martial arts students and teachers of the San Francisco Bay Area. In the experiment, he placed a styrofoam cup on the ground, and I asked the students to try to pick it up while Dr. Yu projected his ch'i on the cup.

It was an odd scene. A student would approach the cup, try to grasp it, and suddenly fall back. One of the most expert martial artists in the group could get no nearer than two feet from the cup. At last it was my turn. Dr. Yu was standing about five feet away from me at the time. With great determination I walked toward the cup and tried to pick it up with both hands. I was sure I could do it. But when my hands were about six inches from the cup, I suddenly felt as if I were holding two strong magnets and trying to force them together. My hands felt pushed apart from the inside, almost as if they had been blown apart by an explosive force. The force was so strong and so surprising that it knocked me off balance, and, like the others, I fell back several steps. The experience was amazing to me because it was the first time I had felt ch'i.

In his later years, Dr. Yu practiced Ch'i Kung almost exclusively for healing. His power was invaluable to the martial arts teachers and students of the area, whose damaged knees and shoulders he treated by projecting his ch'i into the area injured. The ability to project ch'i is rare, but it is a skill that, with training, many people can acquire. For example, Dr. Yang Bao-Tang in Beijing explained his skill as a matter of training and practice. He himself had been trained in Ch'i Kung from an early age by his grandfather: "In China, these sorts of skills were always taught secretly. My grandfather began giving me qigong [Ch'i Kung] after I stopped nursing. In this way, my grandfather projected his Ch'i into my body." Controlling ch'i is difficult, said Dr. Yang, but the ability to do so depends upon nothing more unusual than a good foundation and constant practice. Dr. Yu would have agreed.

A SKEPTICAL VIEW

Illustrations of Ch'i Kung may seem too fantastic to be credible. It may seem that the paralyzed girl could feel the effect of ch'i because she believed she could and wished she could. But then one must also believe that the girl's paralysis was "in her mind" and ask what would give the mind the power to create and maintain such an unpleasant illusion. Skeptics can believe, too, that "suggestion" caused Dr. Yu's students to feel almost painfully shocked when they attempted to pick up the styrofoam cup, but the skeptics must then explain the power of "suggestion" to produce such physical sensations and to spread from the mind of one person to the minds of others.

The following experiment illustrates in terms of Western science how something invisible and immeasurable, like ch'i, might very well control basic processes of the body. In this case, the participants are American doctors, and the immeasurable force is focused attention.

The experiment went like this: Before operating, thirty-nine surgeons had themselves outfitted with electrodes to monitor heartbeat, cuffs to record blood pressure, and masks to measure the amount of oxygen they consumed. They also took various physical and mental tests. While operating, they cut and tied small blood vessels. Physically, this work was no more strenuous than sewing, but the doctors expended as much energy as the average welder or drill press operator at work. Nearly half the group showed a sharp increase in blood pressure, and, on the average, their heartbeats rose to 118 a minute.

(One surgeon's jumped to 155.) A normal resting heart beats about 70 times a minute.[14]

Without any vigorous physical movements, the cardiovascular systems of these doctors had been greatly stimulated. Subjective mental states, like concentrated attention and a sense of the importance of the task, had loaded their systems. Although these surgeons would not say they had altered the flow of their ch'i, some mechanism of equilibrium and balance was profoundly altered by the concentrated attention they brought to their tasks. Mind and body had interacted like a single entity.

Hypnosis, too, reveals close connections between mind and body. An English hypnotherapist specializing in skin reactions studied how hypnotic suggestion works by observing the patient of another hypnotherapist, who had suppressed a woman's intense allergic reactions to pollens. In ten weekly sessions of thirty minutes each, the therapist had placed her under hypnosis, listed her usual symptoms, and told her she would be free from them.

During treatment, pollen extracts were applied to the woman's arm and leg. Some welts appeared, but only on her leg. The allergic reaction had been suppressed in the upper part of her body, where the symptoms of her allergy, now inhibited by hypnotic suggestion, naturally appeared. Further tests showed that while local chemical releases were occurring wherever the pollen had been placed, the capillaries on the woman's arms were not dilating: "This made sense," the researchers agreed, "since the capillaries are controlled by the brain, whereas the chemical response is not."[15] Applying the theory of ch'i, the mind's intention had gained control of the flow of ch'i and had manipulated it to heal the upper part of the woman's body.

All of us agree that the mind exercises a profound influence upon the body. If asked to explain what had happened to the doctors whose heart rates increased, we would agree that they experienced "stress." But what is stress? What explains this response to challenges of all sorts—the changes in breathing, the fast-beating heart, the increasing blood pressure? Applying the concept of ch'i to stress, we might understand it this way: just as a tourniquet can turn off the flow of blood, so can physical or mental events block the flow of ch'i. When the body tenses, it "turns off" the circulation of ch'i and reduces the body's equilibrium. When the tension relaxes, the flow of ch'i continues, and the body "cools down," its various functions returning to a balanced state.

The theory also explains why stress is damaging: when the flow of ch'i is blocked, some cells of the body do not function properly. Over time, this local malfunction will hamper the body's process of self-repair, a process that helps to keep illness from beginning. Although tension followed by relaxation does not threaten health, residual tension, tension that continues after the body has performed the physical or mental task it has geared up to do, can permanently impede the circulation of ch'i, creating stress dangerous to health.

However the process works, in China in 1986[16] there were 26 Ch'i Kung clinics where doctors claimed success in treating high blood pressure, motion sickness, some heart ailments, certain forms of paralysis, and some gastrointestinal, respiratory, and neurological disorders. Today there are many more.

EXERCISING CH'I

That the human being is a microcosm of the universe was the view held in the West before Newton and Descartes. Then, the universe was thought to be composed of four elements—earth, water, air, and fire—and human beings were believed to be made up of the same elements in the form of four "humors." Disease was explained as resulting from an imbalance among the humors, and doctors administered purges or prescribed diets to regulate surplus or deficiency. Unlike Western medicine, which came to accept a mechanical model of the body, traditional Chinese medicine has continued to emphasize harmony and balance or equilibrium.

According to the tenets of traditional Chinese medicine, to maintain the body's equilibrium one should exercise not only the muscles but also the ch'i. The Chinese character for "strength" combines the words for ch'i and muscle power.

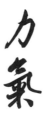

Muscular power alone is not strength; muscles need the inner strength of the body's vital energy.

While exercise can help regulate the flow of ch'i, the exercise must be the right kind. The flow can be regulated only when movement is combined with relaxation and conscious mental guidance. Because T'ai Chi teaches you to seek a certain state of mind while you move, it is sometimes called "a meditation in motion." In China the more common description of T'ai Chi is "internal exercise." This is a more accurate way of explaining what T'ai Chi is about. It means, simply: when you practice T'ai Chi, you use your intention to direct your motion. The movements of T'ai Chi and the focused thought accompanying them exercise the body's ch'i by prompting its flow and exercise the organs of the body by keeping the ch'i flowing through them.

From another perspective, you exercise ch'i simply by not blocking its flow, by *letting* it circulate naturally. The slow-paced, thought-directed movements of T'ai Chi are designed for that purpose: they "unkink the hose" so that the ch'i can flow unimpeded. When you practice the movements this will happen naturally. You need only cooperate with nature. As the philosopher Lao Tzu says, "Nature is simple. It is great because it is simple."

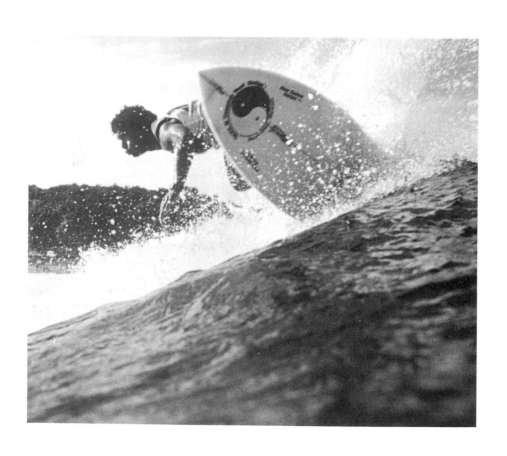

THE BASIC PRINCIPLE OF T'AI CHI: YIN-YANG BALANCE

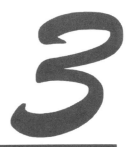

All distinctions appear as opposites.
And opposites are never alone.
They take their meaning from each other.
They complete each other.
We know is *by* is not *and* is not
by is.
Difficult and easy,
Long and short,
High and low,
Loud and soft,
Before and after—
Each takes its meaning from the other.

Lao Tzu, *Tao Teh King*[1]

T'ai Chi or the Absolute is the originator of two equal and opposite principles: the Yin and the Yang; that is, the conserving or replenishing principle, and the activating or spending principle. Whenever there is motion, they separate; whenever there is motionlessness, they recombine.

Wang Tsung-Yueh[2]

To understand how (and why) T'ai Chi Ch'uan works, you need to put the concept of ch'i, discussed in the previous chapter, together with the concepts of yin and yang.

Translated literally, yin means "cloudy" and yang means "sunny." Yin is soft and yang is hard; yin is moist, yang is dry. Yin is empty; yang is full. Sometimes yin and yang are defined as feminine and masculine, a misleading definition because it encourages the belief that things are permanently labeled either yin or yang. In fact, the same thing may be either yin or yang depending upon its relationship to something else. For example, "the roof of a house is yang (up) relative to the ground, but yin (down) relative to the stars."[3]

The divided or yin-yang circle is a symbol of nature for the Chinese philosophers known as Taoists.

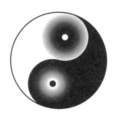

It is a descriptive symbol because everything in nature is composed of a yin element and a yang element. It is also a normative symbol because the health and wholeness of everything in the universe depends upon the "oneness" of the relationship between these yin and yang elements. The more natural this relationship is, the more these elements form one whole, and the better the health and wholeness of animals, plants, or people.

The state of balance between yin and yang elements is dynamic, constantly changing. In humans, this shifting balance of yin and yang is essential to health, for it is the changes in the relationship between yin and yang that keep the body's energy or ch'i flowing freely.

The movements of T'ai Chi Ch'uan embody the dynamic relationship between yin and yang. They are based upon shifting the body's weight to create a continuous intermingling of yin states and yang states. In most movements, either one leg or the other bears the body's weight. The leg bearing the weight is the yang or "solid" leg, while the other, nonweight-bearing leg is "hollow" or yin. Inhalation (yin) and exhalation (yang) also illustrate these principles. That is why T'ai Chi Ch'uan emphasizes smooth, continuous, even breathing. The posture of T'ai Chi Ch'uan, too, encompasses yin and yang: the relaxation of the body—the relaxed abdomen, the relaxed shoulders— is yin; the obvious firmness of the leg is yang. One's attitude also reflects a balance of yin and yang: intention, the inner concentration on the movements, is yin; attention, the monitoring of their accurate physical execution, is yang.

These apparent opposites are one. Everything in nature and every movement in T'ai Chi Ch'uan has a firm side and a soft side, an empty aspect and a solid one. These differences, yin and yang, are revealed when things move or change, but when things are at rest, yin and yang become indistinguishable.

T'ai Chi, then, is an art of self-control achieved and expressed through the balancing of yin and yang. (See Figure 3-1.) Students learn to keep their balance through a continuous series of opposing changes. Both physically and mentally, your center remains stable, like the hub of a moving wheel, even as you pass through the changes of yin to yang and yang to yin.

INTENTION BALANCES ATTENTION

Alert your spirit like a cat ready to surprise a mouse.

Wu Yu-Hsiang, commentary on the Thirteen Movements[4]

First in the mind, then in the body.

A T'ai Chi proverb

Not long ago, researchers in San Francisco, California, ingeniously revealed how the brain gets ready for a task. By studying electrical waves, they showed that the brain does not proceed step-by-step with one item at a time, like a computer following a program. Rather, it activates a whole network of connections, setting up a new network for every task, no matter how familiar the task may be or how similar to a task just performed. During a fraction of a second the brain "sets itself up and forms a new model of what it expects, even for a very stereotyped task."[5] If the set-up is wrong, the response is more often wrong than right.

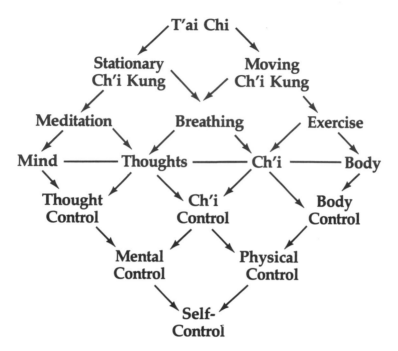

Figure 3-1

This figure shows the dynamic of yin-yang balance. The right side of the diamond follows the yang (or more definite) elements of T'ai Chi. The left side follows the yin (or more indefinite) elements. Reading across the diamond from right to left or left to right shows how the yin elements affect the yang elements and how the yang elements affect the yin elements, in short, how these apparent opposites become one.

What this means is that very often we succeed or fail even before we act. "Many of our errors," says Alan S. Gevins of EEG Systems Laboratory in San Francisco, "are, in a sense, predetermined by a failure to concentrate properly during the split-second before we see or hear something."[6]

THE INTENTIONAL BRAIN

The brain responds to our purposes or intentions. This characteristic, called feedback, allows animals and humans (even plants) to adjust aim to result. A basketball player who misses the first free throw resets his estimate of how much force is required. His body responds with minute muscular readjustments, and on the second throw the basketball sinks perfectly through the hoop. This happens because the brain is neurologically wired to send messages of intention outward as well as to receive information:

> There are two contrasting brain systems: an analytic one which dissects the environment into units of information, and which works, so to say, upward; and an intentional one which uses that information to affect the environment, and works, we may say, downward. The first system is causal; the second is purposive. Definite areas in the fore-brain underlie each of these functions, the analytic and the intentional.[7]

The classic commentators on T'ai Chi placed great emphasis on intention or purpose:

> The movement from [the] feet upward through the legs to the waist should always be fully coordinated. When confusion of movement occurs the cause is to be found in the waist or the legs. Nevertheless, the prime mover is the mind, not anything outside.[8]

Purpose makes the difference between a master and a student, because intention controls inner strength, or ch'i, and puts it to the best use.

Intention not only controls and coordinates movement; intentional thought also has the power to direct ch'i into every part of the body: "Be calm and steady in steering the ch'i with the mind. The least crevice must suffice for passage."[9] Thus intention can increase strength.

The timing of the movements of T'ai Chi allows a guiding intention to precede each movement. T'ai Chi is done slowly because, if the movements became too rapid, they would get ahead of the thought. The movements would then become mechanical or meaningless, confused, and disordered. Then, too, if the movements became rapid, the focus of attention would become spotty as one's thoughts went leaping from part of one movement to part of the next. The flow of ch'i would then become spotty also. Lack of a guiding intention can break the desirable fluidity of movement and interrupt the flow of ch'i. Even worse, no intention at all is like sleepwalking.

The key to thinking while moving lies within you, in the kinesthetic sense. Your thinking or intention has to do with this internal sense, for example, with shifting your weight from one leg to the other or with turning your body or bringing up your arms. Your thought models the movement you intend to make. Especially, your thought models the changes of weight that make your legs "hollow" or "solid," the changes that create yin-yang balance.

A MOVING MEDITATION

When students are told that they must guide their movements and their ch'i by using their minds, many are puzzled. Some connect this lesson with the experience of meditation, especially if they have heard T'ai Chi called "a moving meditation." This idea is a good place to begin, if we define meditation in a T'ai Chi way. Think of meditating as "alert global attention and intention," as thinking and feeling at the same time. As with meditation, you do not think of anything outside yourself as you practice. Especially, you do not go over worries or the details of problems or the duties of the day. If particular thoughts come into your mind, you don't get drawn into them. Instead, you let them fade or "run off," like water from a roof. You should pay attention only to yourself and what you are doing.

A key to monitoring what you are doing is to follow your breathing. The aim is simple: just keep breathing regularly. Let exhalation follow inhalation and inhalation follow exhalation smoothly, without breaks and pauses.

But still students ask, "Where should I focus my thoughts?" The answer is, don't "focus" your thoughts. Think about everything that you are doing. Think about the whole system. In practicing T'ai Chi, you do not focus narrowly on a point but pay attention to a process: what you intend, how it happens, and how it feels. (See Figure 3-2.)

It is the constant linking of movement and thought that so greatly improves students' concentration. Many of our students have found that T'ai Chi helps them to play their favorite sports by increasing their ability to concentrate. Because they have practiced guiding movements with their thoughts while monitoring their breathing and relaxation, these skills come naturally in moments of pressure. One student, a photographer, writes:

> I've played tennis for about twenty years, but since I started practicing T'ai Chi, my focus is much better. I see nothing but the ball—my body does what it's already learned to make the shot.
>
> My partner and I won the mixed doubles tournament at SRI International [a research firm in Menlo Park, California], and I didn't even know the score! During the tournament, whenever I began to choke, I would almost assume the meditation stance and quiet myself immediately.
>
> Also, the last time I had my blood pressure taken, I found it was higher than usual. I asked the nurse to take it again. I then "T'ai Chi quieted" myself and in 30 seconds both readings had dropped, one by 6 points.[10]

What is most remarkable here is that this student did not need to fully assume a particular T'ai Chi posture in order to become calm and relaxed. She needed to *think* about that posture and to *think* about becoming calm. As an early commentator explains, the movements of T'ai Chi are so much directed by the mind and subordinated to it that the thought *is* the movement:

> Up or down,
> front or back,
> left or right, are all the same.
> These are all *Yi* [thoughts] and not external.[11]

Another student, a 34-year-old woman who plays catcher on a softball team, found her movements responsive to her thoughts under highly challenging conditions:

Throughout the two years I have been "playing" [practicing] T'ai Chi, I have continued to discover benefits from regular practice of the exercise. I am an active woman and enjoy participating in all kinds of sports. Swimming, golf, and softball are my favorites.

In the first softball season after I began to practice T'ai Chi, I noticed surprising physical and mental improvements in my performance. In the past, as each new season came around, I had noticed that it took my arms, legs, and shoulders more and more time to recover from the aches and pains that I thought it was necessary to suffer through at the beginning of every season. Since the team I play for does not believe much in practices, I was apprehensive in May 1985—six or seven weeks after I had begun to learn T'ai Chi—when we started the season cold. I was not looking forward to playing two games as catcher without having attended even one practice. To my pleasant surprise, the day-after stiffness I'd come to expect was simply not there. I am sure I can attribute this change to the significant strengthening of the body's muscles, especially the leg muscles, that occurs with practicing T'ai Chi.

Other changes I experienced were even more surprising. Later that same season, perhaps three months after I had begun T'ai Chi, I was involved in a dramatic play at the plate. An opposing player, a big fellow, hit a solid triple, which he tried to stretch into a home run. As this fellow was rounding third for home, I remember blocking the plate in a very low, solid stance. I remember turning towards right field and watching the seams of the ball rotate on a low, hard, accurate throw to me at the plate. In one motion, I gently caught this wonderful throw and turned to make the tag.

Now the base runner, I'm sure, was thinking that his hard slide would take out this woman catcher, but he didn't have a chance. As I put a tag on him, his momentum toward me and the plate was completely redirected, and he ended up in a big dust cloud several feet away. As my team cheered, my opponent sat for a moment in a daze. He didn't know what had hit him, nor did I until the following T'ai Chi class when I put it all together— the concentration on the throw, the lowered center of gravity, the ease in turning and making the tag—this was what T'ai Chi was all about.[12]

This is exactly what T'ai Chi is about. When your thoughts direct your movements and focus your vital energy, then muscle power

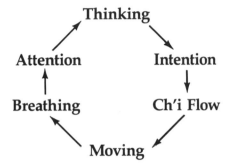

Figure 3-2
This figure illustrates the process of T'ai Chi thought. The right side of the circle shows how intention guides movement. The left side of the circle shows how attention monitors the effects of movement.

combines with ch'i energy. And *then*, as generations of masters have told their students, "Four ounces deflect a thousand pounds."

SOFTNESS BALANCES HARDNESS: A CHILD'S APPROACH TO STRESS

Be gentle and soft.
At birth, we are soft.
Anyone can push us.
We cannot even stand,
Yet we have a whole life ahead of us.
At death, we are hard and tough,
Yet we cannot live for even a minute longer.
All living things
Are soft while they live
But hard and tough after death.
Then gentle is better than tough,
And soft is better than hard.

Lao Tzu, *Tao Teh King*[13]

The vitality of children has inspired parents and grandparents, philosophers and poets. "He who is intelligent is like a little child," wrote Lao Tzu, "his vitality is intact." Children possess almost magical powers of resilience. The "miracle babies" of the Mexico City earthquake, who were found in hospital rubble after many days without food or water, have developed as normal children. When ordinary accidents occur, the speed with which children's bones knit and their cuts heal is the envy of older people.

Thinking about children helps us to understand ourselves as adults. Although children, like adults, feel stress during painful or unpleasant experiences, they quickly throw it off and regain their ability to enjoy life. Unlike them, we adults carry worry around with us—and fear, anger, resentment, and other unpleasant emotions filling us with stress and tension. These tensions emerge in physical symptoms, sometimes causing us to be irritable toward others, and sometimes even affecting our health and recovery power. If we could let go of yesterday's tensions, we might find happiness flowing back into us.

As modern medicine teaches us, tension threatens vitality by literally hardening the body against itself. For example, if tension becomes chronic, the blood vessels lose their resilience. As a leading expert in psychophysiological medicine, Dr. Emmett Miller, explains:

> Any time you are feeling afraid, worried, or "under pressure," you are likely to have an elevated blood pressure. Usually, your blood pressure falls rapidly to normal as soon as you leave the situation that is creating these feelings. This rapid fall of blood pressure back to normal is a property of healthy blood vessels that allows them to maintain adaptive flexibility. As stressful situations grow more and more frequent and as we grow older, the accumulation of unrelieved tension causes the blood vessels throughout the body to become permanently constricted. This constriction of the blood vessels produces greater and greater resistance to blood flow. Imagine trying to blow out a candle through a soft rubber tube. If you begin to constrict the tube by pinching it, you will find that more and more pressure is required for the same amount of air to reach the candle. In the same way, when blood vessels become more and more constricted, a higher blood pressure is needed to pump the blood through the blood vessels, and more work must be done by the heart. The diseases resulting from hypertension and this stress on the heart are many—strokes, heart attacks, kidney disease, angina pectoris, cerebral hemorrhage, and arteriosclerosis, to name a few.[14]

Fortunately, though, as Dr. Miller goes on to explain, our problems come not so much from stress as from *unrelieved* stress. It is chronic stress that leads to serious diseases, as well as to "minor" ailments like depressions and backaches, migraine headaches and upset stomachs, and to the loss of our birthright of happiness. If we discharge stress regularly, we need not fear it. If we act like Lao Tzu's intelligent person who is like a child, we will find ways to throw off tension through play.

Children play simple games. Their favorite games reflect the way they find pleasure simply in existing—in running, balancing, and moving. Knowing how to be vital like a child means knowing how to find pleasure and relaxation in such basic physical experiences.

In many ways T'ai Chi is like a child's game. The common Chinese expression for practicing T'ai Chi Ch'uan is "playing with T'ai Chi." T'ai Chi feels like play in part because it offers no external goals. The philosopher Immanuel Kant once defined a work of art as an entity that is "purposive without purpose." So it is with T'ai Chi. You aim to perform the movements well, to breathe smoothly, and to relax as you move. That's it: you score no points, record no times, and defeat no one. Yet you feel a strong sense of purpose as you move through the beautifully designed forms.

The legend of T'ai Chi's origin is a fable about tension and relaxation, hardness and softness. As the story goes, a sage, Chang San-Feng, watched a battle between a crane and a snake. The crane was attacking the snake fiercely with its beak. Each time the bird struck, the snake, with the slightest motion, slipped out of reach. While the crane struck its beak on the ground, injuring itself with the force of its own blow, the snake, with the same yielding movement, moved away from the blow and gathered its strength to strike back at the bird. Soon the crane was losing the fight. Then it changed strategy. Instead of hitting at the snake with sharp blows from its beak, the bird spread its wings and gently placed them over the snake, which could no longer move out of reach. Softness and yielding, Chang San-Feng saw, were superior to hardness and force.

This lesson is repeated often by the Taoist philosopher Lao Tzu. Water, for example, illustrates the power of softness.

> Nothing is weaker than water.
> Yet for attacking what is hard and tough
> Nothing surpasses it,
> Nothing equals it.
> What is weak overcomes what is strong.
> What yields overcomes what resists.
> This principle is known to everyone.
> Yet few use it
> And profit from it in practice.
>
> Tao Teh King[15]

NOT ONLY CHILDREN ARE YOUNG

In the traditional lore of T'ai Chi as a martial art, the ability to control softness and yielding is often given as a key reason why an old master of T'ai Chi can overcome a young fighter. A classic treatise on T'ai Chi describes the superiority of T'ai Chi as a skill that overcomes force, a skill illustrated by age defeating youth:

There are many misleading ways of teaching the art of boxing.

Although differing from one another, they all share one common principle and that is: The stronger in brute force necessarily overwhelms the weaker. The slow-moving hand seeks in vain to dodge the fast-moving.

But these are only empirical formulae which cannot take the place of true knowledge based on philosophical research. It is quite obvious that preponderance of physical strength alone does not explain the toppling of one thousand pounds with a trigger force of merely four ounces. He is not relying on speed when an old man successfully defends himself against the simultaneous attacks of many youthful opponents. Something more than arithmetic is involved.[16]

This favorite theme is often fleshed out with stories of old men whose soft movements turn aside the attacks of younger men. Our own T'ai Chi teacher, Kuo Lien-Ying, had his version of this experience. In his youth, Kuo had learned a martial art in which speed and hardness were the goals, only to be defeated by a very old master who knew how to become soft. Here is an account of Master Kuo's meeting with the man who became his T'ai Chi master, together with a testimony to Kuo's own power, by one of his students who had spent many years practicing "hard" martial arts like karate:

Kuo worked as a body guard and would often travel with goods or money which needed protection. While outside Peking one day, he discovered that a great T'ai Chi master called Wang, then 104 years old, lived nearby. Kuo, anxious to know more about T'ai Chi and to prove himself, confronted the famous master and challenged him. Master Wang effortlessly neutralized all of Kuo's attacks. Kuo bowed before his superior and became his student.

On my last day of formal training with him, Master Kuo demonstrated his skills to me and asked me to attack him. He easily outmaneuvered me and deflected all my attacks. He would either circumvent my blocks and land light punches on my body, or with an effortless touch, send me sailing into a wall. With all my "hard" style training, I could neither elude him nor attack him. His soft relaxed system worked. At this time, Kuo was in his late 80's and I was in my late 20's.[17]

Softness is also playfulness. Resilience, flexibility, and humor go together. Master Kuo was loved by his students for his playfulness. In spite of his great skill, he carried himself modestly, without formality or pretension. Young people and children attended his classes, held outdoors in Portsmouth Square in San Francisco. He sometimes amused them by eating watermelon, seeds and all, or by staring into the sun without blinking, or by eating garlic cloves whole. Among T'ai Chi masters, a childlike warmth and direct simplicity are common. In *Encounters with Qi* David Eisenberg draws an affectionate portrait of Old Chang, who taught T'ai Chi to students at the Institute of Traditional Chinese Medicine in Beijing:

> He was as playful and fit at sixty as a child of eight. Unlike most Chinese men, Old Chang was totally bald. "I have a shiny egg for a head," he would say in his self-deprecating style. "Thank goodness I am already married!" He wore baggy blue cotton sweatsuits over white thermal long johns. His belt was a common piece of cord. This short, raggedly clothed man had the muscles of a gymnast, the grace of a dancer, and the balance of a cat. No ordinary cat, though. Old Chang was a human lion with unmatched power and agility.[18]

By "playing with T'ai Chi" you keep your vitality intact, let go your worries, and become resilient again like a child.

Learning the softness of T'ai Chi may save your life. If that seems too dramatic, in spite of what doctors tell us about heart disease and high blood pressure, then consider this story. Near Stafford, Virginia, William Heaser, 42, stopped on an interstate highway to help a motorist whose car had crashed just ahead of him. As he was opening the door of the wrecked car, he saw another car speeding toward him, so he leaped over the guard rail to escape it. Unfortunately, Heaser failed to notice that he had driven onto a bridge:

> I jumped over the barrier, thinking I would land on the ground on the other side, but I just kept on falling. My first impression was, "What a great feeling!" It must have been the same sensation skydivers get. In the next second, I knew I was in big trouble. I was saying to myself, "I'm not supposed to be enjoying something like this."
>
> Then, I remembered what my brother, Richard, told me when he was in jump training with the Green Berets. "Just before you land, you exhale all your air and just go limp." I did that. I don't remember hitting the trees, but it hurt real bad when I hit the ground.[19]

Heaser had fallen 115 feet. He ruptured his spleen and punctured a lung. His jaw, wrist, finger, ribs, shoulder, and all the bones in his left leg were broken. A month later he was recuperating at home. How could this be? By luck, no doubt—and by the power of softness, relaxation, and control.

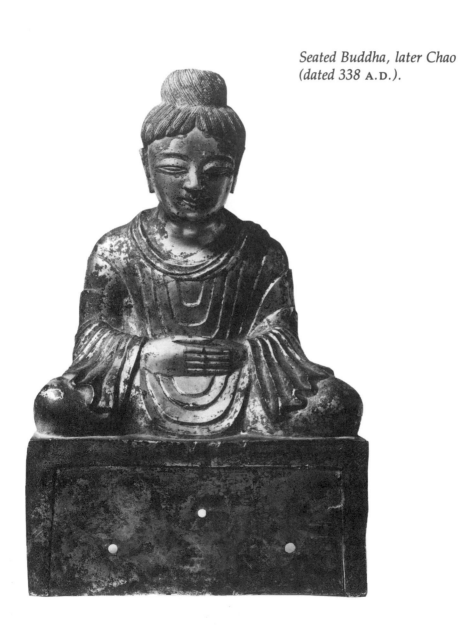

Seated Buddha, later Chao (dated 338 A.D.).

PREPARING FOR T'AI CHI WITH CH'I KUNG

4

In the first three chapters of this book, you have learned the theory behind Ch'i Kung and T'ai Chi. You are now ready to learn the Ch'i Kung exercises and to prepare for your practice of the T'ai Chi forms, and so to begin your own practice of these ancient arts.

Ch'i Kung has a history even longer than that of the martial arts. Written records have been found of Ch'i Kung practices dated as early as 1100 B.C. These were used as self-healing exercises, and they were adapted to fit the philosophies and special needs of many groups—Confucianists, Taoists, Buddhists, herbalists, acupuncturists, and others.

Ch'i Kung exercises were taught in secret. In particular, they became the secret training exercises of the Hsing Yi school of martial arts. Like T'ai Chi Ch'uan, Hsing Yi begins its modern history in the seventeenth century and by tradition traces its roots to the Sung Dynasty, which ended in 1279. Hsing Yi martial artists had an almost supernatural goal: to develop the power to project the body's energy, and thus to immobilize an opponent without touching him.

Like T'ai Chi, Ch'i Kung was set aside in revolutionary China, though it was still practiced by popular artists who performed amazing feats: breaking stones with their heads, supporting heavy baskets hung on their ears by a rope, bending steel bars with a single kick, and so on. In recent years it has become a subject for medical research. David Eisenberg, the American doctor who was introduced to T'ai Chi on his trip to China in 1979–1980, became fascinated by Ch'i Kung masters: in Beijing he watched a master make the tassels of a hanging lamp (and the lamp itself) move without touching them; at the Shanghai Institute of Traditional Chinese Medicine he saw another master turn a dart hanging on a string, again without touching it; on a second trip to China, in 1983, he watched as a master lit a 5-foot, 40-watt fluorescent bulb by slapping and rubbing it with his hands.[1] Though these curious demonstrations of the external application of ch'i were prompted by courtesy to a visitor and were not part of a medical program, the use of Ch'i Kung in medical treatments is a subject of research at the institutes and at all major hospitals.

CH'I KUNG EXERCISES

The exercises have two aims. One is to relax the body in order to open it to an unobstructed flow of ch'i. The other is to use the mind to direct the flow. The means to these ends are simple: smooth, even breathing; relaxation; and mental intention and attention accompanied, in some cases, by local massage.

Breathing, in addition to being a means of directing the ch'i flow, is a source of ch'i and is the most important source, for we breathe many times each minute, while we eat only a few times a day. Our lives are composed of many cycles—waking and sleeping, eating and fasting, moving and resting—but the cycle nearest to each minute of our lives is the cycle of breath. We can live without food for days or even weeks, but stop our breath and we are soon gone.

Breathing naturally, which you should do during all the movements described in this book, moves the ch'i. Thinking consciously, as you will be directed to do by the instructions for the movements, also moves it. Both together mean that the vital force of the body is stimulated by the practice of Ch'i Kung.

HOW TO USE THESE EXERCISES

Use Exercises 2 through 5 as warm-up exercises before each session of T'ai Chi. These exercises improve the circulation of ch'i in the areas stimulated by the exercise's local massage: lower back, hips, ankles, and knees. Use Exercise 1, *The Sitting Meditation*, to practice feeling the movement of ch'i and to calm your mind. It is useful for beginning or ending the day or for replenishing your energy when you take a break from work.

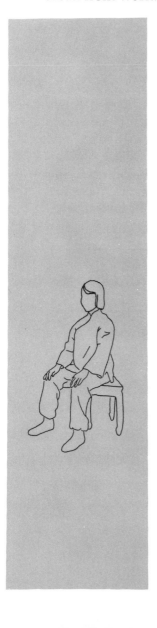

CH'I KUNG WARM-UP 1: THE SITTING MEDITATION

The Sitting Meditation enhances the flow of the body's energy from your arms to your legs. It also helps you to feel that flow as a sensation of warmth. For this exercise, you need ten minutes without interruption and the right place to sit. The seat must be firm, level, and the right height.

What is the right height? The height at which your feet rest flat on the floor and your thighs are level and parallel to the floor. If the seat is too low, your thighs will slope up toward your knees; if too high, your thighs will slope down. As you sit, your thighs and legs should be like two sides of a square box. If a straight chair is too low or too high, a coffee table or a stool may be what you need.

1-A Sit erect, with shoulders and abdomen relaxed. Place knees slightly apart, on a line with hips. Place feet directly below knees, pointing straight ahead, toes even. Rest palms, flat, lightly on knees. Close your eyes, and let your attention remain unfocused, directed globally toward your whole body.

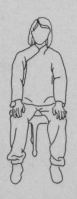

1-B (Front view) If thoughts, words, or images come into your mind, let them pass. Treat them like stray dogs following you along a street. Pay no attention to them and let them wander away. Sit quietly for ten minutes.

Checking Yourself

- Thighs level.
- Feet parallel, toes even.
- Shoulders relaxed.
- Abdomen relaxed.
- Attention global.

Sometime during the ten minutes you may feel warmer, and you may feel a tingling sensation. Your knees may feel a penetrating warmth where your palms lie against them. The exercise is beneficial whether you feel such sensations or not, so don't try to make them happen. Keep your attention unfocused and relaxed and breathe regularly.

CH'I KUNG WARM-UP 2: CIRCLING THE MIDDLE (BACK EXERCISE)

This exercise encourages energy to flow by gently stirring its source, the body's center, giving the body an internal massage. Your palms channel energy through sensitive points in the lower back (acupuncture points). Enjoy the movement. Too many adults think exercise means "No pain, no gain." These exercises feel like play.

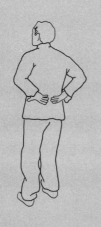

Relax your shoulders; let them drop. (Habitually hunched shoulders can help bring on headaches.)

2-A Stand with feet apart, on a line with hips, feet parallel, toes even, weight evenly balanced, knees slightly bent, facing straight ahead. Relax your abdomen. Bend your knees slightly, and distribute your weight evenly. Place palms on the lower back, just above the waist, fingertips on each side of the spine, not touching.

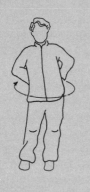

2-B Push your abdomen gently forward and circle it *slowly* around to the right twelve times.

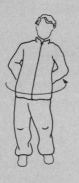

2-C Push your abdomen gently forward and circle it around *slowly* to the left twelve times.

Checking Yourself

- Weight evenly balanced, toes even.
- Knees slightly bent.
- Shoulders relaxed.
- Abdomen relaxed.
- Hands on lower back, fingers not touching.

Repeat until you have done two dozen circles. Breathe smoothly and slowly.

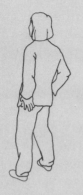

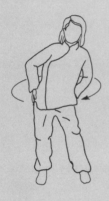

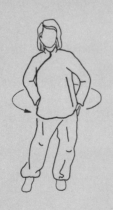

CH'I KUNG WARM-UP 3: HIP STRENGTHENING

In this exercise your palms channel energy through the hip joint while slow rotation gives the joint a gentle massage.

3-A Stand with feet apart, in line with hips. Place your palms flat, fingers down, lightly on hip joints. Relax hands and fingers. Relax abdomen and shoulders. Take a few steps forward and back. If your palms are over the joint, you will feel it move.

3-B Slowly and gently, swing the right hip out to the right and circle it to the back, ending where you began. (The circle will be small, and flat on the front side.)

3-C Repeat with the left hip.

Checking Yourself

- Feet apart, toes even.
- Weight evenly balanced.
- Palms on hip joints.
- Knees slightly bent.
- Swing right, circle back.
- Swing left, circle back.

Breathe slowly and smoothly. Sometimes students concentrate so hard on doing a movement that they forget to breathe. Smooth, regular breathing is an essential part of Ch'i Kung.

As the joint grows more flexible you may feel or hear a popping in the hip joint as you circle it. This is a sign of flexibility. Don't, however, force the joint. Always circle gently and slowly.

Do twelve circles each way until you have done two dozen altogether.

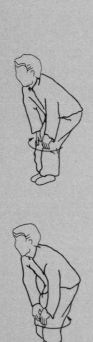

In this exercise your palms channel energy into your knees while the slow rotation gently massages the joint. The Greeks believed that the strength of the body lay in the knees, and some doctors tell their patients, "Your knees are a second heart." This exercise helps to keep knees flexible. Your posture and the circling motion will also flex and gently exercise your ankles.

4-A Place the palms of your hands lightly over your knees, feet straight ahead, toes even. Raise your head and look straight ahead. Bend your knees slightly and circle both knees slowly to the right, keeping knees close together but not touching.

4-B Circle both knees slowly to the left, keeping feet close together but not touching.

Checking Yourself

- Knees bent, weight evenly balanced.
- Feet straight ahead, toes even.
- Palms over knees.
- Eyes straight ahead.
- Circle knees right.
- Circle knees left.

Do twelve circles each way. (Fewer circles should be done if knees have been injured.)

Keep the circles slow and even, all at the same rate of speed.

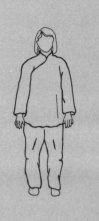

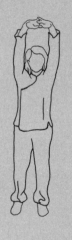

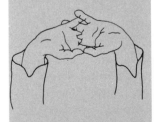

CH'I KUNG WARM-UP 5: UPWARD STRETCH AND LOOSENING

Stretching and bending from side to side are part of many calisthenic routines. Thought to have originated in Sweden in the eighteenth century, such routines were introduced there in a treatise by a French Jesuit missionary to China.[2]

5-A Stand with feet parallel, not touching, pointing straight ahead, weight evenly distributed, toes even, knees slightly bent. Relax abdomen.

5-B Lace your fingers in front of you, palms down. With fingers interlaced, stretch your arms over your head, palms up.

See close-up of hands in position 5-B.

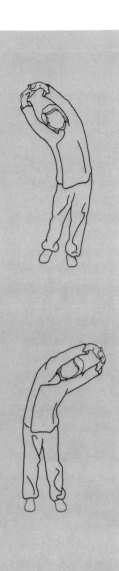

5-C Bend gently and slowly to right side, pushing palms up to stretch your left side.

5-D Bend gently and slowly to left side, pushing palms up to stretch your right side.

Checking Yourself

- ■ Feet apart, parallel, weight even.
- ■ Lace fingers.
- ■ Stretch arms, palms up.
- ■ Bend right.
- ■ Bend left.

Bend to each side six times.

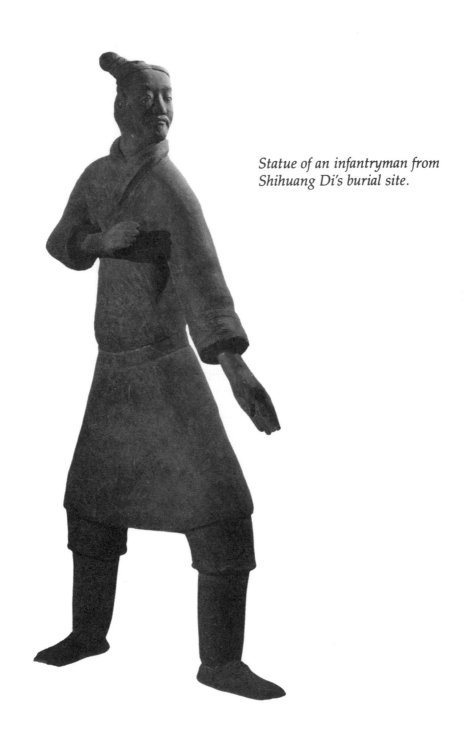

Statue of an infantryman from Shihuang Di's burial site.

T'AI CHI CH'UAN 5

HISTORY

Just when T'ai Chi Ch'uan was first practiced no one knows. The formulation of the system is traditionally assigned to Chang San-Feng of Wutang Mountain, who, though he may well be legendary, is said to have lived from about 1279 to 1368 A.D. So great is the prestige of T'ai Chi that according to some legends Chang San-Feng also discovered the secret of rejuvenation and lived 250 years. Certainly, T'ai Chi Ch'uan is an ancient martial art. Its name means "global and optimal way of fighting with the fist," and a life-sized terra-cotta figure from the Ch'in dynasty (221–210 B.C.) shows a foot soldier stepping forward in a posture resembling a T'ai Chi movement.[1]

The roots of T'ai Chi, however, lie in the philosophy and medicine of Taoism, associated with Lao Tzu, who is said to have been born in 604 B.C. He, too, may be a legendary figure: his name means simply "the Ancient." The Taoists were philosopher-scientists who believed in the power and bounty of nature. To these sages, wisdom lay in following nature, yielding to nature, and doing nothing to oppose nature. This was the True Way, the Path, or Tao, and it led to health, happiness, and long life.

The Taoists were China's earliest physicians. The origins of traditional Chinese medicine lie in their explorations. Traditional medicine owes to them the beginnings of its immense pharmacopoeia of herbal treatments and also its knowledge of the body's sensitive pressure points. The Taoists called their study of the natural ways to preserve youth and health and to prolong life "internal alchemy." Their philosopher's stone was a youthful and ageless maturity.

The system of exercise associated with the Taoists' teachings and practice is "internal" exercise. Expressing their Taoist belief in yielding to nature, the system emphasizes soft, natural movements; smooth, effortless breaths; a stance firmly grounded on the earth; and conscious mental attention to guide and unify the process. Movements begin in the mind and activate the whole body from within, just as nature itself is set in harmonious motion by an inner force.

Students are guided by images from nature:

Be still as a mountain.
Walk like a cat.
Move like the clouds, so slowly that no one can see
   the changes as you move.

A painting from the Han dynasty (c. 168 B.C.) shows many figures exercising in T'ai Chi-like postures named for various animals, among them the crane, the dragon, and the monkey, animals whose names are still attached to movements today.[2] Movements have also been named for the tiger, the rooster, and the horse.

The very name of these exercises is rooted in the Taoists' natural philosophy. Literally, *T'ai Chi* means "supreme ultimate" or "global optimal," or, translated more expansively, "the global state of perfection." In Taoist philosophy, T'ai Chi is a concept denoting a stage in the evolution of the cosmos, a point of harmonious balance between a state of emptiness (the void that existed before creation) and a state of unstable fullness, of matter in dynamic motion.

The third word in the name, *Ch'uan*, means fighting without a weapon. Translated into English, this becomes, rather misleadingly, "boxing." As a system of patterned movements designed to improve strength, flexibility, coordination, and endurance, T'ai Chi is like other forms of exercise. It is unlike most other forms of exercise, however, in its mental component, designed to improve concentration and self-control by training the student to focus thought on a series of movements while preserving a sense of continuity from one movement to the next, as if the whole series were one single movement. This mental concentration helps to account for the sense of effortless fluidity that students of T'ai Chi come to prize.

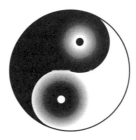

The symbol for the state of T'ai Chi is a circle divided into yin (or emptiness) and yang (or fullness). Within each division is a small circle. Within yin, this circle represents yang; within yang, yin. This illustrates that yin and yang interact with each other in an endless succession of changes. T'ai Chi is the whole that encompasses cosmic "shifts of weight" between the poles of empty, weightless yin and full, solid yang, while combining inhaling yin and exhaling yang in the natural pattern of breathing.

The exercises based upon the concept of T'ai Chi teach a student how to achieve a state of dynamic equilibrium, a state of relaxed wholeness encompassing emptiness and fullness through change and movement. In this state, the student is balanced (sometimes briefly motionless), yet always preparing to move; inwardly calm, with a spirit composed and still, yet ready in an instant to call upon a stream of energy as powerful as a cracking whip. In the days of hand-to-hand combat, a fighter trained in T'ai Chi Ch'uan knew the "supreme-ultimate globally optimal way to fight without a weapon." The philosopher, however, valued T'ai Chi for something more: its power to bring a student into optimal harmony with the great patterns of nature, to reduce disharmony or friction between the individual and the cosmos, and so to promote healing, health, and long life.

T'AI CHI CH'UAN IN MODERN TIMES

Because of its great reputation both as a martial art and as a way to healthy longevity, T'ai Chi in old China was treated as a valuable possession. Family clans held it within the family. Great masters took few disciples and trained them in secret. Not surprisingly, then, the recorded history of T'ai Chi is of a comparatively recent date.

The modern history of T'ai Chi begins in the seventeenth century with the Ch'en family, a dynasty of masters from whom descend the chief modern styles of T'ai Chi—Ch'en, Yang, and Wu. The most famous of the Yang family masters was Yang Lu-Shan (1800–1873), whose renown followed from both his skill and his independent nature. Yang broke with tradition by accepting students from outside the family clan. Consequently, his style of T'ai Chi became the best known of all the variations upon the traditional forms. It is still the most popular style in China and elsewhere.

The style of T'ai Chi in this book descends from Yang Lu-Shan through just four generations: Yang Lu-Shan; Yang's elder son, Pan-Hou (1837–1892); Wang Cheu-Yeu (1810–1924); Kuo Lien-Ying (1897–1984). Master Yang Pan-Hou was T'ai Chi instructor to the imperial family (and only to the family) at the end of the Ching dynasty. Wang Cheu-Yeu was his secret student and successor as grand master. Kuo Lien-Ying was chosen by Wang Cheu-Yeu to succeed him. Thus, Master Kuo, our teacher, was the fourth-generation grand master in the Yang school of T'ai Chi Ch'uan.

Although Yang Lu-Shan taught T'ai Chi outside his clan, he did not open his classes to the public. He, too, practiced an elite art. The nationalist revolution in China, however, changed the history of T'ai Chi. Post-revolutionary China had no place for the traditions and secrets of the great clans. Thus, the practice of T'ai Chi became more openly known. At the same time, the prestige of T'ai Chi suffered owing to its association with the feudal past. Because of the communist revolution in China, many T'ai Chi masters, like my teacher Kuo Lien-Ying, who had formerly been a congressman from Inner Mongolia, left China. T'ai Chi became widely dispersed abroad.

THE PRESTIGE OF T'AI CHI

During the Cultural Revolution (1966–1976), T'ai Chi suffered severely from its association with the elitism of ancient China. In public, it was neither taught nor practiced. Now, however, T'ai Chi Ch'uan has been restored to its place as a national treasure, like landscape painting or calligraphy. It is practiced daily in cities and villages; throughout the country, schools teach the skill. In North China, Beijing alone offers over 160 centers. In 1979–1980, when the American doctor, David Eisenberg, studied traditional medicine at the Beijing Institute of Traditional Chinese Medicine, a valued member of the staff was "Old Chang," the institute's T'ai Chi master. It has been estimated that some 400,000 people have studied in such centers in Canton (Guanzhou) in South China.

HOW TO LEARN THE T'AI CHI MOVEMENTS

The T'ai Chi movements are divided here into fifteen lessons, designed to take fifteen minutes each to learn. The illustrations will show you how to learn arm and leg movements separately for each movement and then how to combine them in a continuous motion. To establish the linkage needed for continuity, the directions for every new movement begin with the end of the preceding movement. This overlapping will teach you how to connect the movements in sequence. Following each set of illustrations is a checklist to help you with the basic elements of the movement.

Begin your daily practice by loosening up with the Ch'i Kung exercises in Chapter 4. Then do the T'ai Chi movements in this chapter. After you have practiced sufficiently to learn the movements, doing the Ch'i Kung warm-ups once and the set of T'ai Chi movements three times will take about ten or fifteen minutes. All twelve T'ai Chi movements can be done, slowly, in less than three minutes. If you add the sitting meditation, your practice will take twenty to twenty-five minutes.

Although the Yang system we teach includes sixty-four movements, the first twelve movements contain the basic theory and practice of the full set. The benefits of practice are not tied to a particular number of forms: one of the nineteenth-century treatises on T'ai Chi is called "Insights into the Practice of the Thirteen Postures."[3] The twelve movements presented here, then, are close to a classic number of forms. Furthermore, enhanced by our method and coupled with the practice of Ch'i Kung exercises, these movements will answer your needs for good health, peace of mind, and relief of stress.

The first T'ai Chi movement you will learn is called The Grand T'ai Chi Movement. Although it is the last movement in the series, we teach it first because it is most often the movement where students can first feel ch'i move through their bodies. It offers the essential benefits of both T'ai Chi and Ch'i Kung—calming, healing, and strengthening. We ask that you end every practice session with it.

GUIDE TO DAILY PRACTICE

The following things remain constant whenever you practice:

> **Orientation:** Place yourself within a rectangle that measures about 7 x 5 feet, and face a long wall. All movements will be oriented within this rectangle.

> **Relaxation:** Always relax abdomen and shoulders and bend knees slightly. Let shoulders drop; keep knees loose, not locked. Hands are relaxed, palms open, fingers slightly apart.

> **Breathing:** Breathe smoothly and regularly. Let movements regulate breathing. Pay attention to breathing; don't hold your breath.

> **Erect posture:** Keep torso erect and look straight ahead. (Don't lean to one side, bend forward or back, or look at the floor.)

> **Symmetry:** The right leg stays on the right side of the body, the left leg on the left. As you step forward or backward, don't let your feet cross the center line of your body.

> **Shifting weight:** Your weight is usually on one leg at a time. We call the weight-bearing leg the "solid" leg and the free or non-weight-bearing leg the "hollow" leg.

> **Balanced weight:** Sometimes your weight is on both legs. We then say "Weight even" or "Sit in the middle." "Sit in the middle"

means bending your knees slightly and letting your legs support your body as though you are sitting on the edge of a stool with your back straight.

Pace: Move at the same slow pace through every form and movement, as if you were unwinding a single, fragile thread of silk. This image comes from the traditional writers, and the thread they have in mind is a single filament of a silkworm's cocoon.

Intention: Be mindful of each movement and, when you have learned a movement, let your mind lead you through it; think before and as you move. Sometimes we say "Use your intention." This means "Let your mind direct your action."

Attention: Be aware of what you are doing—your movement, breathing, relaxation, and distribution of weight. Monitor the whole process.

Clothing: Wear loose-fitting clothes and soft-soled, flexible, flat-heeled shoes.

Practice: Each day practice all the movements you have learned up to that date. Practice them in their sequence several times. Do not practice immediately after eating.

NOTE ON LEARNING THE MOVEMENTS

As you read the instructions and follow the corresponding illustrations for each lesson, you will find that each lesson begins with a front view, unless otherwise noted. Follow the instructions in regard to the direction you are to face while doing the exercise.

Once you've mastered a movement, follow the instructions at the end of the lesson to perform in sequence all movements learned up to that point. When you have mastered all the lessons and have performed them in order, you will have completed a counter-clockwise circle.

The photographs of Master Lee in the beginning of each lesson show you the beginning and ending positions for each movement.

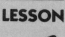

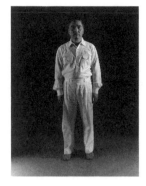

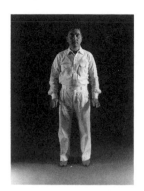

THE GETTING READY STANCE AND THE GRAND T'AI CHI MOVEMENT

The Getting Ready Stance

When you do this stance you prepare your mind and body for all T'ai Chi movements. While in this balanced position you relax your body and calm your mind. Use your mental intention to "lower" your energy to your abdomen and legs and let all your weight sink down to your legs. Do this before every movement.

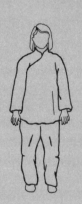

- Stand up. Have your feet parallel and placed at the width of your shoulders. Keep your weight evenly balanced on both legs with your knees loose. Relax arms at sides, slightly away from your body.
- Breathe evenly, with your whole body relaxed. This will mentally prepare you for T'ai Chi.
- Quietly feel that your weight is going down to your feet.

The Grand T'ai Chi Movement

This movement usually comes at the end of a sequence of T'ai Chi movements. Because of its effectiveness in moving ch'i freely to every part of the body, we have been teaching our students to do it at the end of each new movement they learn. When you learn all twelve movements, this one will take its place as the last. To perform this movement the Ch'i Kung way, pay attention to your breathing. As you begin to learn the movement make sure you breathe naturally. Once you have mastered the movement use your mental intention to "breathe with your entire body" as you raise your arms. As you lower your arms in front of your body, pay attention to the feeling of the ch'i flow. Take as many breaths as you find necessary during the movement. This movement uses the palms of the hands to direct the flow of ch'i evenly to every part of the body.

While practicing this movement, keep your entire body relaxed. You should feel a wave of warmth flowing from head to feet, a tingling sensation in the palms, and the sensation of a column of warm air in front of your chest. Because this movement helps reduce stress and promote healing, it is used to end each session of practice. It is usually through this movement that our students feel the flow of ch'i for the first time. We hope this will happen to you. Even if you don't feel the ch'i flow, however, you will feel good all over—from top to bottom, inside and out, physically and mentally. Any time you feel that you are under stress, simply get up and do the *Grand Movement* a few times. It will help reduce stress and rejuvenate your body immediately. As we often tell our students, if all you have is thirty seconds, this is the movement you should practice. If you prefer, you may close your eyes when you do it.

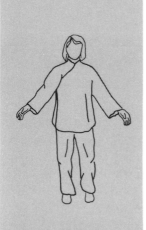

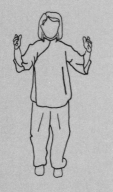

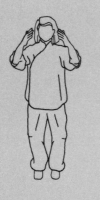

Learning the Grand T'ai Chi Movement

1-A Stand in the *Getting Ready Stance*. Bend knees slightly and sweep arms out and up in an arc, forming a large circle.

1-B Bring arms up to shoulder height, elbows slightly bent, palms facing each other at chest height.

1-C Raise both hands to face height, arms in a circle, palms in, not touching, fingers apart.

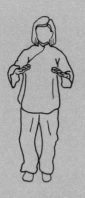

1-D Slowly lower hands in front of your body, arms in a circle, palms turning down. Straighten knees.

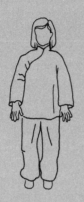

1-E Return arms to sides slowly, with palms down.

Checking Yourself

- Move arms at same pace and keep both arms at the same height.
- Weight evenly distributed on both legs.
- Feet parallel.
- Knees slightly bent.
- Breathe smoothly with whole body relaxed.
- Look straight ahead.

Practice the *Grand Movement* four times slowly.

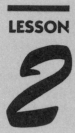

2

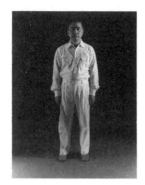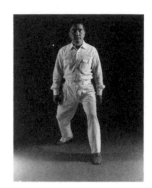

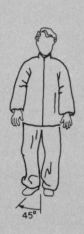

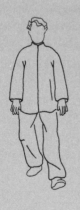

THE ONE-LEG SOLID STANCE AND THE TWO-LEG SOLID STANCE

These two basic stances illustrate the shifting of weight that takes place with most of the T'ai Chi movements. These stances stimulate your ch'i flow, strengthen the muscles in your legs and lower back, and improve your body's balance, posture, and stability. After practicing these movements, shake each leg gently to be sure that your muscles are loose.

Right-Leg Solid Stance

2-A   Face any direction in the *Getting Ready Stance*. Bend knees slightly and turn right foot out 45 degrees.

2-B   Shift weight to right leg. Move left foot forward, heel down, toe up (45 degrees off floor), knee straight. Feel that your weight is going down to your right foot.

Checking Yourself

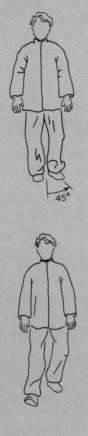

- If right leg does not feel comfortable, bend it less.
- If left leg does not feel hollow, move it closer to you.
- If you do not feel balanced, be sure that your left leg is directly in front of your hip.

Left-Leg Solid Stance

2-C Face any direction in the *Getting Ready Stance*. Bend knees slightly and turn left foot out 45 degrees.

2-D Shift weight to left leg. Move right foot forward, heel down, toe up (45 degrees off floor), knee straight. Feel that your weight is going down to your left foot.

Checking Yourself

- If left leg does not feel comfortable, bend it less.
- If right leg does not feel hollow, move it closer to you.
- If you do not feel balanced, be sure that your right leg is directly in front of your hip.

First do the *Right-Leg Solid Stance* four times (stand as long as you are comfortable). Shake your legs gently after each stance. Repeat the same with the *Left-Leg Solid Stance*. Do this sequence four times.

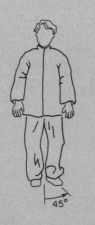

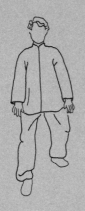

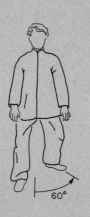

The Two-Leg Solid Stance

This is the basic stance to develop the feeling of stability and centering. It is the leg stance which is used in movements where the arms are pushing or punching. As you push or punch, do it with your whole body. Mentally make the connection between your legs and arms. If you relax your legs and "sit" on them evenly, they become firm and solidly grounded. You can feel how firm your legs are just by pressing them with your finger.

The *Two-Leg Solid Stance* should be done first with right leg forward, following the instructions below. Then perform the mirror image of the exercise, beginning with your left leg forward.

2-E Start with the *Getting Ready Stance*, then shift weight to left leg, turning left foot out 45 degrees. Make the right leg hollow, lifting foot slightly off the floor.

2-F Step forward with right leg, foot directly in front of your hip, toes pointing straight.

2-G Turn left foot out a little more (60 degrees). Bend knees evenly, sitting in the middle, weight on both legs.

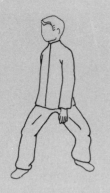

See side view of 2-G.

Checking Yourself

- Body faces forward.
- The knee of the front foot is bent forward slightly, and the knee of the back foot bent out slightly.
- If you do not feel comfortable, make sure that your body is centered, your knees are bent evenly, one foot is directly in front of your hip, and the other foot is turned out 60 degrees.
- Shoulders and hips are facing forward, with arms relaxed along sides.
- Look straight ahead.
- Knees and legs are relaxed.

Stand as long as you are comfortable. Repeat the stance with the left leg forward. Do this sequence of stances four times, shaking your legs gently after each stance.

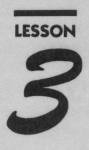

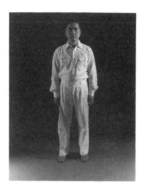

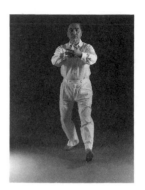

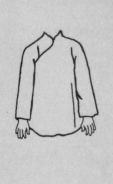

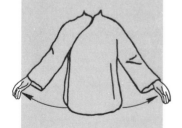

PAY RESPECT TO MANKIND

This first movement of T'ai Chi is a symbolic gesture to show respect for mankind. To perform this movement the Ch'i Kung way, you should pay attention to your breathing while you do the movement. After you have mastered it, as you raise your arms, pay attention to inhalation. As you bring your hands together to form a circle, pay attention to exhalation. While doing the movement, take as many breaths as you need to feel comfortable and relaxed. The ch'i flow will be different in each leg, depending on whether the leg is hollow or solid.

Arm Movement

3-A Arms at sides, palms in, shoulders loose.

3-B Slowly sweep both arms up and out in an arc.

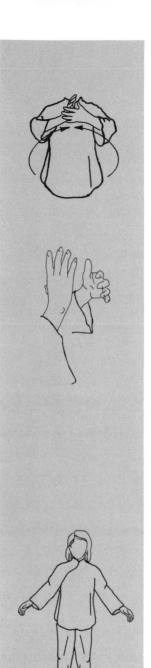

3-C Form a circle with arms in front of chest, left hand ahead, right hand behind. Right hand bisects left palm, not touching.

See close-up of hand position for 3-C.

Checking Yourself

- Body faces front wall.
- Right hand bisects left.
- Shoulders are down, relaxed.
- Elbows at equal height.
- Look forward and breathe evenly.

Repeat the arm sequence (3-A to 3-C) four times slowly or until you have memorized the sequence.

Leg Movement

3-D Face front wall. Stand in the *Getting Ready Stance*. Bend knees slightly. Turn right foot out (45 degrees).

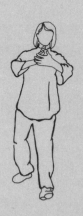

3-E Shift weight to right leg. Move left foot forward, heel down, toe up (45 degrees off floor), knee straight but not locked. Feel weight going down only to your right leg.

Checking Yourself

- Body faces front wall.
- If right leg does not feel comfortable, bend it less.
- If left leg does not feel hollow, move it closer to you.
- If you do not feel balanced, make sure that your left leg is directly in front of your hip.

Repeat the leg sequence (3-D and 3-E) four times or until you have memorized it.

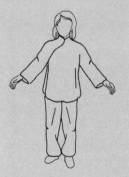

Combining Arm and Leg Movements

3-F Bend knees slightly. Stand in the *Getting Ready Stance*, facing front wall. Turn right foot out (45 degrees). Shift weight to right leg. Slowly sweep arms up and out.

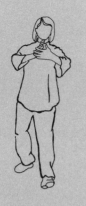

3-G Slowly move left foot forward, heel down, toe up (45 degrees), and raise arms to form circle in front of chest.

Checking Yourself

- Body faces front wall.
- Right leg solid, left leg hollow.
- Right foot turns out (45 degrees).
- Left foot rests on heel, toe up (45 degrees off floor).
- If right leg does not feel comfortable, bend it less.
- If left leg does not feel hollow, move it closer to you.
- If you do not feel balanced, be sure that your left leg is directly in front of your hip.
- Breathe evenly, with whole body relaxed.

To end the movement, bring left heel next to right heel, and turn right foot parallel to left foot. Now do the *Grand Movement*.

Repeat 3-F and 3-G four times or until you have memorized them. Shake your legs gently at the end of each.

Practice from the beginning (3-F to 3-G) and end with the *Grand Movement* (1-A through 1-E) several times. Shake your legs gently at the end of each repetition.

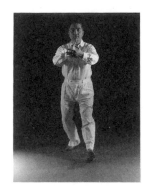 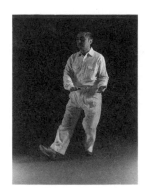

GRASP BIRD'S TAIL (FIRST HALF)

The first half of the movement symbolizes pulling someone's arm to the left as if grasping a bird's tail.

In the first half of the movement, as you start to lower your arms, pay attention to inhalation. After your hands have been lowered, pay attention to exhalation. Your intention is to bring your energy closer to you. Your attention is directed to relaxing your wrists, arms, and shoulders. As you lower both hands to the left side (grasping the bird's tail), you can feel your ch'i between your palms.

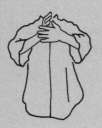

Arm Movement

4-A Place arms in the final position of *Pay Respect to Mankind* (3-G).

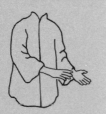

4-B Pull both hands slowly toward left side of body.

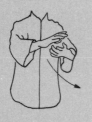

4-C Lower hands to waist height, left side, elbows bent, right palm down, left palm up, right hand slightly in front of and above left hand.

Checking Yourself

- Hands at waist height, palms open with left palm up, right palm down.
- Fingers apart and pointing toward front wall.
- Elbows bent.
- Wrists and shoulders loose.

Repeat the sequence of movements (4-A to 4-C) four times or until you have memorized it.

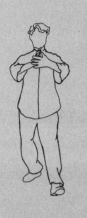

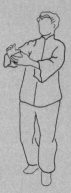

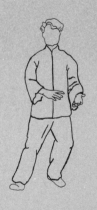

Leg Movement

4-D Stand in the final leg position of *Pay Respect to Mankind* (3-G), facing front wall.

4-E Turn body toward right corner and begin to step backward by bringing left heel back to right heel, keeping left foot close to floor with left toe pointed straight ahead, weight on right leg.

4-F Step back on left foot. Shift weight to left leg, knee bent, toes out (45 degrees). Right leg is hollow and rests on heel, toes up (45 degrees off floor).

Checking Yourself

- Body faces right corner.
- If left leg does not feel comfortable, bend it less.
- If right leg does not feel hollow, move it closer to you.
- If you do not feel balanced, make sure that your right leg is directly in front of your hip.

Repeat 4-D through 4-F four times or until you have memorized them. Shake your legs gently after each.

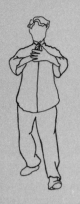

Combining Arm and Leg Movements

4-G Stand in the final position of *Pay Respect to Mankind* (3-G), facing front wall.

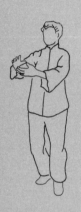

4-H Turn body toward the right corner, keeping arms in circle. Begin to step back with left heel, keeping foot close to the floor and toes pointed toward front wall.

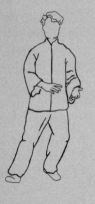

4-I Step back on left foot, shifting weight to left leg. Pull both hands slowly to left side, right palm down, left palm up. Weight on left leg, right leg hollow. Right foot rests on heel, toes up (45 degrees off floor).

Checking Yourself

- Begin facing front wall; end facing right corner.
- Begin with weight on right leg; end with weight on left leg.
- If left leg does not feel comfortable, bend it less.
- If right leg does not feel hollow, move it closer to you.
- If you do not feel balanced, make sure that your right leg is directly in front of your hip.
- Hands at waist height, palms open, with left palm up, right palm down.
- Fingers apart and pointing toward front wall.
- Elbows bent.
- Wrists and shoulders loose.
- Breathe evenly, with whole body relaxed.

To end the movement, bring right heel next to left heel and turn left foot parallel to right foot. Repeat the sequence (4-G through 4-I) and do the *Grand Movement* (1-A through 1-E) four times slowly. Shake your legs gently after each movement.

Practice from beginning to end all the movements you have learned—*Pay Respect to Mankind* and *Grasp Bird's Tail, First Half*—and end by doing the *Grand Movement* at least twice. Shake your legs gently at the end of each sequence.

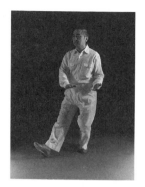
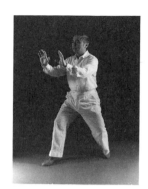

GRASP BIRD'S TAIL (SECOND HALF)

This movement symbolizes pushing someone's body away in front of you.

In the second half of the *Grasp Bird's Tail* movement, when you start to bring up your hands, pay attention to inhalation. If you use your intention to gather your ch'i, you should feel a "ball" of warm air between your palms and your body. If you keep your arms and legs relaxed, as you push forward you should feel your ch'i as a wave of warmth flowing from your body to your palms and your feet.

Arm Movement

5-A   Place arms in the final position of *Grasp Bird's Tail, First Half* (4-I).

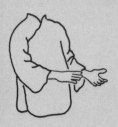

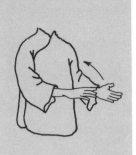

5-B Raise hands slowly, keeping elbows bent.

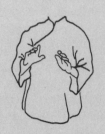

5-C Bring hands in front of chest, palms out.

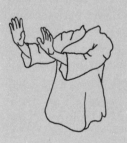

5-D Push forward (with both hands).

Checking the Movement

■ Body faces right corner.
■ Arms almost fully extended (elbows slightly bent), both hands the same distance from body.

Repeat 5-A through 5-D four times or until you have memorized the sequence.

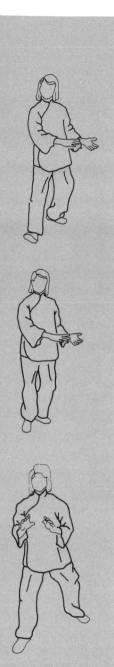

Leg Movement

5-E   Stand in the final position of *Grasp Bird's Tail, First Half* (4-F), facing right corner.

5-F   Bring right heel to left heel.

5-G   Step forward with right foot directly in front of your hip, toes pointing straight ahead.

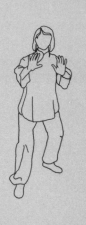

5-H Turn left foot out a little more (to 60 degrees). Bend knees evenly, sitting in the middle, weight evenly distributed on both legs.

Repeat movements 5-E through 5-H four times or until you have memorized them. Shake your legs gently after each movement.

Checking Yourself

- Body faces right corner.
- If you do not feel comfortable, make sure that your body is centered, your knees are bent evenly, and your right foot is directly in front of your hip.

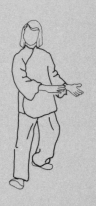

Combining Arm and Leg Movements

5-I Stand in the final position of *Grasp Bird's Tail, First Half* (4-I), facing right corner.

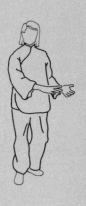

5-J Bring right heel to left, slowly raising hands, elbows bent.

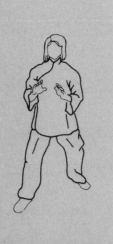

5-K Step forward with right foot, bringing hands to chest, palms facing away from chest.

5-L Sit in the middle, turning left foot out (60 degrees), and push forward, knees bent slightly.

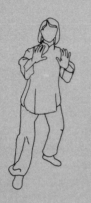

Checking Yourself

■ Body faces right front corner, weight even, both legs solid, body upright.
■ Breathe evenly, with whole body relaxed, mind calm, making sure that you are comfortable.

To finish the movement, bring right heel back to left heel, feet parallel, heels not touching. Now do the *Grand Movement* (1-A through 1-E).

Repeat the sequence (5-I to 5-L) four times slowly and end with the *Grand Movement*. Shake your legs gently after each movement.

Practice from beginning to end the movements you have learned (3-F through 5-L) and end by doing the *Grand Movement* (1-A through 1-E) at least twice. Shake your legs gently at the end of each sequence.

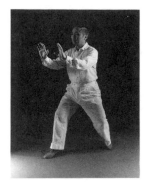
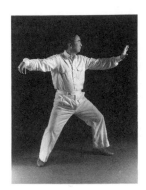

LESSON 6

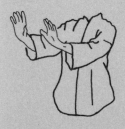

SINGLE WHIP

This movement symbolizes pushing an opponent with an outstretched left arm. As you bring your hands closer to your chest (first half of the movement), pay attention to inhalation. If you use your intention to gather your ch'i, you should feel a "ball" of warm air in front of your body. As you move your arms outward in an arc (the second half of this movement), pay attention to your exhalation.

Arm Movement (First Half)

6-A Place arms in the last position of *Grasp Bird's Tail* (5-L), facing right corner.

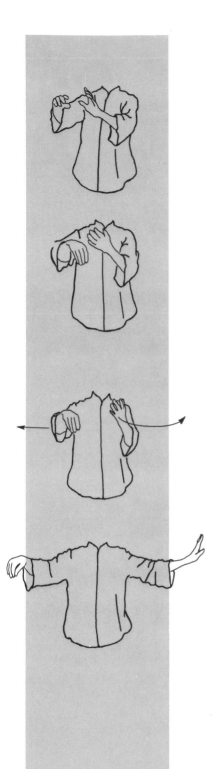

6-B Bend elbows, bringing hands closer to chest.

6-C Turn left palm toward chest and right palm down, wrist loose. Bring right thumb and fingers down together, like a beak. Let right wrist droop.

Checking Yourself

- Elbows bent, arms not touching body.
- Elbows at same height.
- Relax right wrist.

Arm Movement (Second Half)

6-D Move arms outward in an arc without raising elbows. Turn left palm toward chest, keep right hand in beak.

6-E When arms are almost fully extended, turn left palm out and push gently toward left wall. Let right arm curve slightly, wrist loose.

Checking Yourself

- Arms almost fully extended, forming a large arc with the shoulders.
- Neck, shoulders, arms, and wrists relaxed.

Repeat the sequence of movements (6-A through 6-E) four times or until you have it memorized.

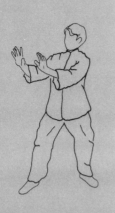

Leg Movement (First Half)

6-F   Stand in final leg position of *Grasp Bird's Tail* (5-L), facing right corner.

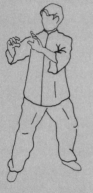

6-G   Turn right foot to face front wall, shifting weight to right leg.

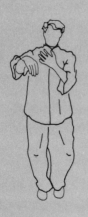

6-H   Bring left toe to right instep.

Checking Yourself

■ Begin facing right corner; end facing front.

■ Shift weight from even distribution on both legs to weight on right leg.

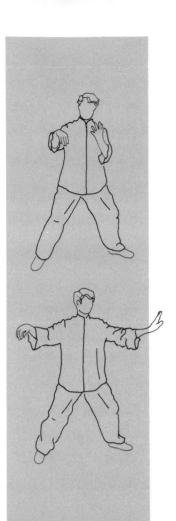

The Leg Movement (Second Half)

6-I Take a step with the left foot toward the left wall. Right foot, not moving, points to front wall. Left foot points to left wall, with left heel in line with the right heel.

6-J Bend knees, sitting in the middle comfortably with weight evenly distributed on both legs.

Checking Yourself

- Begin with right leg solid; end with both legs solid.
- Knees bent evenly.
- Both legs relaxed.

Repeat the sequence of movements 6-F to 6-J four times slowly or until you have it memorized. Shake your legs gently after each.

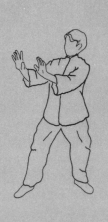

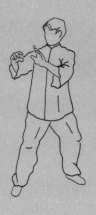

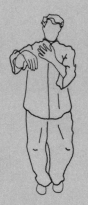

Combining Arm and Leg Movements

6-K Start in the final position of *Grasp Bird's Tail* (5-L), facing the right corner.

6-L Turn right foot to face front wall, shifting weight to right leg. Rotate body to face front wall, bringing arms in front of chest, elbows bent slightly.

6-M Bring left toe parallel to right instep, turning left palm toward face, right palm down, fingers in beak, wrist drooping.

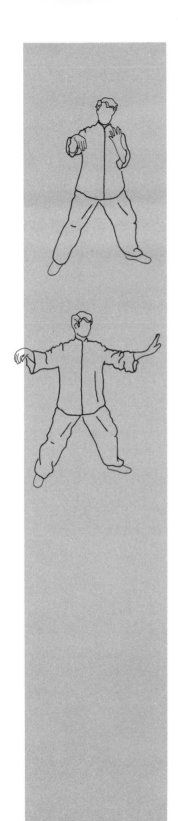

6-N Take a step toward the left wall with left foot, moving arms outward in arc.

6-O When left arm is in front of left shoulder, push forward gently, palm out, turning head to look left. Sit in the middle, weight evenly distributed between legs.

Checking Yourself

- Begin with body facing right corner; end with body facing front wall.
- Shifting weight: begin with both legs solid; shift to right leg solid; end with both legs solid.
- Left foot points to left wall, right foot to front wall.
- Arms are almost fully extended, elbows slightly bent.
- Curve right arm slightly forward.
- If you do not feel comfortable, make sure that your body is centered and your knees are bent evenly.
- Both hands extend equally at the same height.
- Left heel is lined up with your right heel along a line parallel to the front wall.
- Relax your neck, shoulders, arms, and wrists.

To end the movement, turn body toward left wall. Bring right heel to left heel, not touching. Follow with the *Grand Movement.*

Repeat the sequence of movements 6-K to 6-O four times slowly or until you have it memorized. Shake your legs gently after each sequence.

Practice several times from beginning to end all the movements you have learned, starting with *Pay Respect to Mankind* and ending with the *Grand Movement.* Shake your legs gently at the end of each sequence.

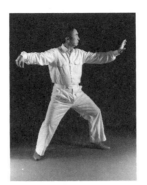 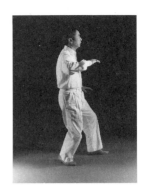

WHITE CRANE SPREADS ITS WINGS

This movement symbolizes striking an opponent with your right elbow. You lift your right elbow gracefully as a bird balancing on one leg and spreading its wings.

In the first part, as you turn your body and move your right foot forward, pay attention to inhalation. Concentrate on bringing your ch'i to the front with your right arm and pushing your ch'i to the floor with your left arm. If you keep your arms and legs relaxed, you can feel a wave of warm air surrounding you that extends from your arms to the floor.

In the second half of this movement, as you step to the side with your right foot, pay attention to exhalation. When you move your right elbow to the side and your left elbow to the rear, you should feel a wave of warm air moving around you from front to back.

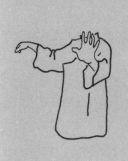

Arm Movement (First Half)

7-A Place arms in the final position of the *Single Whip* movement (6-O).

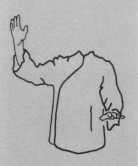

7-B Bend elbows, raising right arm in front of right shoulder, lowering left arm to waist.

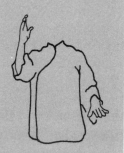

7-C Move right hand forward slightly, edge of hand facing away from body. Push down gently with left hand, keeping hand at waist height, palm down.

Checking Yourself

- ■ Fingers apart.
- ■ Hands and wrists relaxed.
- ■ Left palm at waist level.
- ■ Shoulders relaxed.
- ■ Right elbow down.

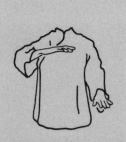

Arm Movement (Second Half)

7-D Move right elbow toward right side, bringing right hand closer to your body. Turn right palm down, chest height, parallel to floor. Move left elbow slightly forward.

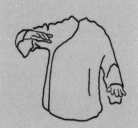

7-E Keeping right arm at chest level, move right elbow to right. Move left elbow slightly to rear, pressing down gently with left hand, waist height.

Checking Yourself

- ■ Right elbow, shoulder height, pointing toward front wall (to your right).
- ■ Right hand in front of chest, fingers not touching.
- ■ Left elbow, pointing toward the rear, slightly away from body.
- ■ Left hand at waist level, palm down, fingers not touching.

Repeat the sequence of movements (7-A to 7-E) four times or until you have memorized them.

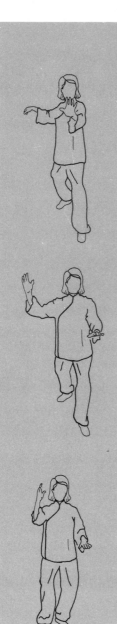

Leg Movement (First Half)

7-F Stand in the final leg position of the *Single Whip* movement (6-O), body facing front wall.

7-G Turn both feet toward left 45 degrees, pivoting on heels, keeping knees bent slightly. Rotate body toward left wall.

7-H Shift weight to left leg. Move right foot forward in line with right hip, ball of foot on floor with heel slightly raised.

Checking Yourself

■ Left leg solid, foot turned out 45 degrees.

■ Right leg hollow, foot parallel to front wall, heel off floor.

■ Right leg on right side of body, foot pointed forward.

■ If left leg does not feel comfortable, bend it less.

■ If right leg does not feel hollow, move it closer to you and lift up the knee slightly.

■ If you do not feel balanced, be sure that your right leg is directly in front of your hip and your left leg is turned out 45 degrees.

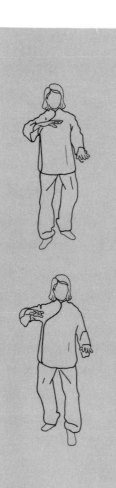

Leg Movement (Second Half)

7-I Begin in position at end of 7-H. Bring right heel to left heel and step to the right, toe pointing out 45 degrees, and shift weight to right leg.

7-J Move left foot forward, pointing straight ahead (toward left wall), resting on ball, heel up, parallel to front wall, left leg hollow.

Checking Yourself

- Face left wall.
- Right leg solid, foot turned out 45 degrees.
- Left leg hollow, foot parallel to front wall, heel off the floor.
- Left leg on left side of body, foot pointed forward.
- If right leg does not feel comfortable, bend it less.
- If left leg does not feel hollow, move it closer to you and lift up the knee slightly.
- If you do not feel balanced, be sure that your left leg is directly in front of your hip and your right foot is turned out 45 degrees.

Repeat the sequence of movements 7-F through 7-J four times or until you have them memorized. Shake your legs gently at the end of each sequence.

Combining Arm and Leg Movements

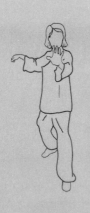

7-K Stand in the final position of the *Single Whip* (6-O), pushing toward the left wall with left arm.

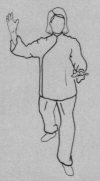

7-L Rotate body to face left wall. Turn both feet to left 45 degrees. Bend elbows, bringing right arm forward, fingers open, palm facing left, lowering left arm to waist, palm down.

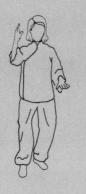

7-M Shift weight to left leg. Begin to step forward with right foot, keeping foot close to the floor. Rest foot on ball, heel slightly up. Move right hand slightly forward, edge of hand facing away from body.

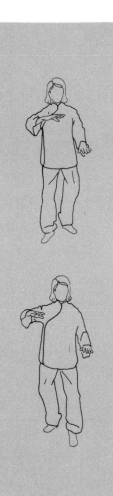

7-N Lower right hand to chest height, palm down. Bring right heel back to left heel and then step to right, shifting weight to right leg, foot turned out 45 degrees.

7-O Push right elbow to right, arm level with chest. Move left foot forward to rest lightly on ball, heel up. Push left elbow back slightly.

Checking Yourself

- Begin facing front; end facing left wall.
- First half: shift weight from both legs solid to left leg solid.
- Second half: shift from left leg solid to right leg solid.
- Check for comfort and balance; adjust leg position if necessary.

To end the movement, bring left heel next to right heel, and turn right foot parallel to left foot. Follow with the *Grand Movement*.

Repeat the sequence four times or until you have it memorized. Shake your legs gently after each sequence.

Now practice all of the movements you have learned, beginning with *Pay Respect to Mankind* and ending with the *Grand Movement*. Do this twice. Shake your legs gently at the end of each sequence.

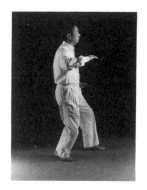 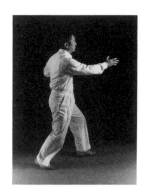

BRUSH KNEES AND TWIST STEP

This movement symbolizes deflecting an opponent to the side. While stepping backward and maintaining a firm balance, you sweep your arms to the side.

In this movement, as you are stepping (when your weight is supported by only one leg), pay attention to inhalation. At the same time, use your intention to bring your ch'i to the side with your palms. At the end of a step backward, pay attention to exhalation. If you keep your arms and legs relaxed, you can feel a wave of warm air moving down to your feet.

Arm Movement

8-A Place arms in the final position of *White Crane Spreads Its Wings* (7-O).

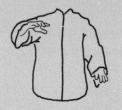

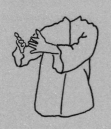

8-B Elbows bent, bring your hands to the right and back slightly, left hand ahead of right, both palms facing right. (Think of right hand as "pulling," left hand as "pushing.")

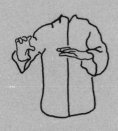

8-C Elbows bent, bring right hand forward and left hand back.

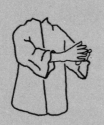

8-D Bring hands to the left and back slightly, right hand ahead of left, both palms facing left. (Think of left hand "pulling," right hand "pushing.")

Checking Yourself

- ■ Face left wall while moving hands; don't turn to either side.
- ■ Hands at same height, fingers parallel to floor, apart.
- ■ One hand six inches ahead of the other, hands a little below shoulder height.
- ■ Hands and wrists relaxed; forward hand "pushes," back hand "pulls."

Repeat the sequence of arm movements (8A to 8D) four times or until you have memorized it.

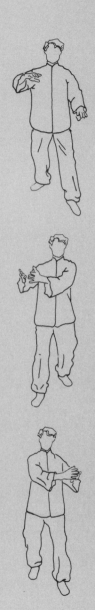

Leg Movement

8-E Stand in the final stance of the *White Crane Spreads Its Wings* (7-O).

8-F Step back on left foot, with toes turned out 30 degrees. Turn right foot in slightly. Sit in the middle; weight even.

8-G Step back on right foot, with toe turned out 30 degrees. Sit in the middle; weight even.

Checking Yourself

- Face left wall.
- Body erect, centered, weight even.
- Knees bent slightly, but loose.
- Both feet turned out 30 degrees at end.
- If you do not feel balanced, make sure that your feet are not crossing the center of your body. Right heel should be on right side, left heel on left side.
- If you do not feel comfortable, make sure that your weight is distributed evenly on both legs. You may need to shift your body either forward or back to redistribute your weight evenly.

Repeat the sequence of movements (8-E to 8-G) four times or until you have it memorized. Shake your legs gently at the end of each sequence.

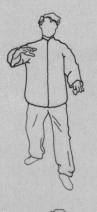

Combining Arm and Leg Movements

8-H Stand in the final position of the *White Crane Spreads Its Wings* (7-O), facing left wall.

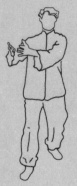

8-I Step back on left foot, turning toe out 30 degrees. Turn right foot in slightly, from 45 to 30 degrees. Sit in the middle; weight even. Elbows bent, push palms to right, just below shoulder height, left hand ahead of right. Move hands back slightly, left hand ahead.

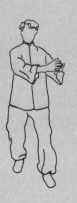

8-J Step back on right foot, turning toe out 30 degrees. Let left foot turn to point left 30 degrees. Sit in the middle; weight even. Elbows bent, push palms to left, just below shoulder height, right hand ahead of left. Move hands back slightly.

Checking Yourself

- Face left wall.
- Step backward: left, right.
- Body erect, weight on one leg when stepping back and weight even when pushing with both hands.
- Check for comfort and balance; adjust body or leg positions if necessary.

To end the movement, bring left heel next to right heel, and turn right foot parallel to left foot. Follow with the *Grand Movement*.

Repeat the sequence (8-H to 8-J) four times, each time ending with the *Grand Movement*. Shake your legs gently after each sequence.

Now practice *all* of the movements you have learned twice and in sequence, beginning with *Pay Respect to Mankind* and ending with the *Grand Movement*. Shake your legs gently at the end of each sequence.

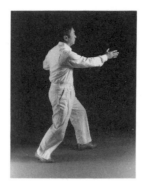
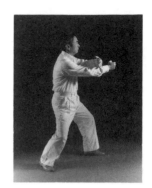

DEFLECT, PARRY, AND PUNCH

This movement symbolizes deflecting some-one's arm to the side with a sweep of the left hand and delivering a punch with the right arm.

In this movement, as you shift your weight to your right leg, pay attention to inhalation. At the same time, use your intention to gather your ch'i with your hands toward your body. As you step forward, pay attention to exhalation. If you keep your arms and legs relaxed, you can feel a wave of warm air moving forward as you punch.

Arm Movement

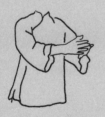

9-A Place arms in the final position of the *Brush Knees and Twist Step* (8-J).

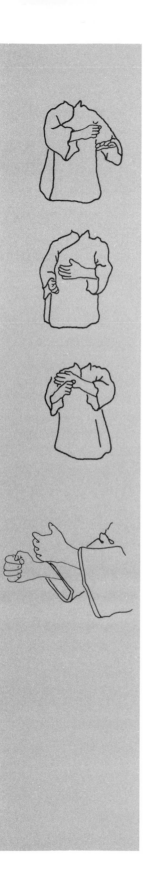

9-B Make a loose fist with your right hand and begin to pull right hand back to right side. Move left hand forward.

9-C Bring right hand down to waist height, knuckles down; sweep left arm, curved at chest height, in front of body, palm in.

9-D With left arm facing body at chest height, palm in, fingers open, punch forward slowly with right hand, rotating fist to left 90 degrees as you punch. (Punch under left arm.)

See close-up of hands in position 9-D.

Checking Yourself

- Face left wall.
- Right fist loose.
- Left arm curved, palm toward you, not touching right arm.
- Punch slowly under left arm, rotating fist to left (from knuckles down to knuckles on right).
- Right arm extended almost fully, with elbow slightly lowered.

Repeat the sequence of movements (9-A to 9-D) four times or until you have memorized it.

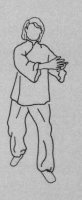

Leg Movement

9-E Stand in the final leg position of *Brush Knees and Twist Step* (8-J).

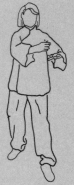

9-F Turn right foot out 45 degrees. Shift weight to right leg.

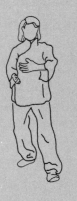

9-G Raise toes of left foot, resting foot on heel. Move heel slightly back, leg straight. Left leg hollow; right leg solid.

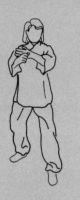

9-H Step forward on left foot, toes pointing straight ahead (toward left wall). Turn right foot out 60 degrees. Bend both knees slightly and distribute weight on legs evenly. Sit in the middle in the *Two-Leg Solid Stance* (2-G).

Checking Yourself

■ Face left wall.
■ Shift weight: first, from even on both legs to right leg (as in the basic right leg solid stance); then, from right leg solid to weight even, both knees bent.
■ If you do not feel comfortable, make sure that your body is centered, your knees are bent evenly, and your left foot is directly in front of your hip.

Repeat the sequence of movements (9-E to 9-H) four times or until you have it memorized. Shake your legs gently at the end of each sequence.

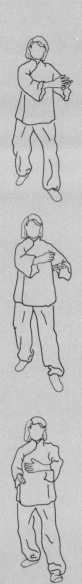

Combining Arm and Leg Movements

9-I   Stand in the final position of *Brush Knees and Twist Step* (8-J).

9-J   Turn right foot out 45 degrees. Start to shift weight to right leg. Make loose fist with right hand and bring left arm forward.

9-K   Shift weight onto right leg. Raise toes on left foot, resting foot on heel. Pull right hand back to waist, knuckles down. At same time, sweep left arm, curved, chest height, palm in, across body.

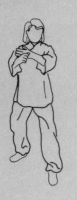

9-L Step forward on left foot and punch forward under left hand, weight even.

Checking Yourself

- Face left wall.
- Shift weight, from even distribution to right leg, and back to even distribution.
- Punch slowly, right fist loose, arms not touching.
- Check for comfort and balance; adjust body or leg positions if necessary.

To end the movement, bring left heel next to right heel, turn right foot parallel to left foot, and do the *Grand Movement*.

Repeat the sequence (9-I to 9-L) and end with the *Grand Movement* four times or until you have it memorized. Shake your legs gently after each sequence.

Then practice twice *all* of the movements you have learned, ending with the *Grand Movement*. Shake your legs gently at the end of each sequence.

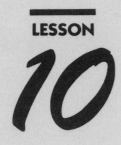
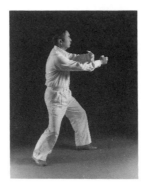 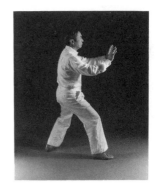

APPARENT CLOSE-UP

In this movement, an apparent pull-back or withdrawal is followed by a smooth push.

As you are shifting your weight to your right leg, pay attention to inhalation. At the same time, use your intention to bring your ch'i in your palms toward your body. If you keep your arms and legs relaxed, you can feel a wave of warm air moving toward you. As you step forward, pay attention to exhalation.

Arm Movement

10-A Place arms in the final position of *Deflect, Parry, and Punch* (9-L).

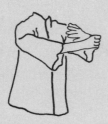

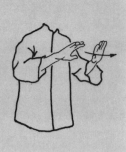

10-B Open right fist and hold palms forward with wrists and hands relaxed. Bring elbows down and close to body. Bring hands in toward chest.

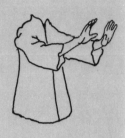

10-C Push palms forward, extending arms and keeping elbows slightly bent.

Checking Yourself

- Face left wall.
- As you pull hands back toward chest, elbows don't touch body.
- As you push forward, arms don't extend fully.

Repeat the sequence of movements (10-A to 10-C) four times or until you have memorized it.

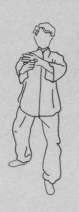

Leg Movement

10-D Stand in the final leg position of *Deflect, Parry, and Punch* (two-leg solid stance, 9-H).

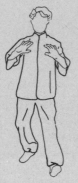

10-E Turn right foot in slightly and shift weight to right leg, raising toes of left foot, resting left foot on heel. Bring heel in toward you until knee becomes straight in the basic right-leg solid stance.

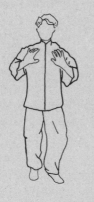

10-F Turn left foot out 45 degrees and step down on it. With weight on left leg, start to step forward with right foot by bringing right heel next to left heel.

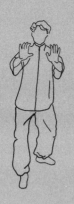

10-G Step forward with right foot and turn left foot out from 45 degrees to 60 degrees. Sit in the middle in the *Two-Leg Solid Stance* (2-G), weight even.

Checking Yourself

■ If you do not feel comfortable, make sure that your body is centered, your knees are bent evenly, and your right foot is directly in front of your hip.

Repeat the sequence of movements (10-D to 10-G) four times or until you have it memorized. Shake your legs gently at the end of each sequence.

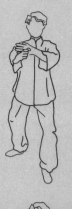

Combining Arm and Leg Movements

10-H Stand in the final position of *Deflect, Parry, and Punch* (9-L).

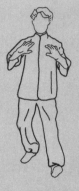

10-I Turn right foot in slightly (to 45 degrees). Shift weight to right leg, raising toes on left foot, bringing left heel back slightly (to make it feel hollow). Pull arms back toward chest, elbows bent, palms out.

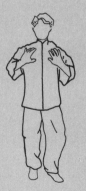

10-J Turn left foot out 45 degrees and step down on it. Shift weight to left leg. Begin to step forward with right foot, keeping foot close to floor and toes pointed straight ahead. Start to push both hands forward.

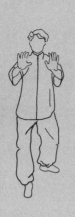

10-K Step forward on right foot to complete the push. Turn left foot out an additional 15 degrees. Weight even, sit in the middle, with knees bent slightly.

Checking Yourself

- Shift weight from right leg to both legs.
- Begin by pulling back, left foot ahead, left leg hollow and right leg solid.
- End by pushing, right foot ahead, weight even.
- Check for comfort and balance, adjust body or leg positions if necessary.

To end the movement, bring left foot parallel to right foot, and do the *Grand Movement*.

Repeat the sequence four times (or until you have it memorized), ending with the *Grand Movement*. Shake your legs gently after each sequence.

Then practice all of the movements you have learned, beginning with *Pay Respect to Mankind*, ending with the *Grand Movement*; complete sequence twice. Shake your legs gently at the end of each sequence.

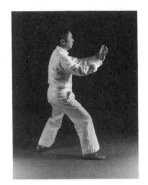 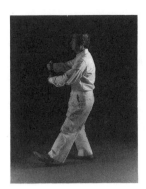

CARRY TIGER TO MOUNTAIN (FIRST HALF)

This movement begins with a turnaround (first half) to stop an attacker from behind, and it continues with a pursuit of the attacker.

In this movement, as you turn around and move your arms to form a circle, pay attention to inhalation. You can feel your ch'i in front of you between your arms. After you turn, pay attention to exhalation.

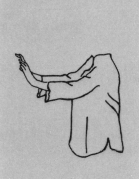

Arm Movement

11-A (Side view.) Place arms in the final position of the *Apparent Close-Up* (10-K).

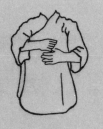

11-B Make a loose fist with right hand; bring both hands toward body, forming a circle with arms, right hand above left. Left palm faces chest; hands do not touch. (When you combine the arm and leg movements for this sequence, you will turn your body toward your left as you pull your hands in toward your chest.)

Checking Yourself

- Begin, arms extended.
- End, arms in circle.
- Keep right fist loose.

Repeat the sequence of movements (11-A to 11-B) four times or until you have memorized it.

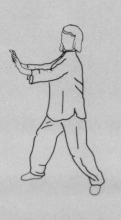

Leg Movement

11-C (Side view.) Stand in the final leg position of the *Apparent Close-Up* (two-leg solid stance), facing left wall (10-K).

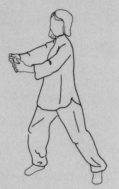

11-D Pivot right foot toward left. Shift weight to right leg, knee bent. Continue to turn to left, pivoting on your right heel.

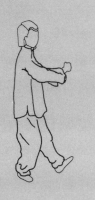

11-E Weight is on your right leg, with your right foot turned out 45 degrees. Lift left heel off the floor and move it forward to align with left hip, toes pointing up 45 degrees from floor, knee straight. Stand in the right foot solid stance.

Checking Yourself

- ■ Pivot on right foot to your left.
- ■ Begin facing left wall, end facing right wall.
- ■ If right leg does not feel comfortable, bend it less.
- ■ If right knee does not feel comfortable, make sure that right foot is turned out 45 degrees.
- ■ If left leg does not feel hollow, move it closer to you.
- ■ If you do not feel balanced, be sure that your left leg is directly in front of your hip at end of sequence.

Repeat the sequence of movements (11-C to 11-E) four times or until you have it memorized. Shake your legs gently at the end of each sequence.

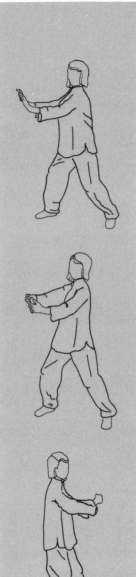

Combining Arm and Leg Movements

11-F Stand in the final position of the *Apparent Close-Up* (10-K), facing left wall.

11-G Pivot on right foot, turning body to left. Shift weight to right foot, making a loose fist with right hand and forming a circle with arms, chest height. Right hand is above left hand, which is open, palm in. Hands do not touch.

11-H Keeping arms in a circle, right fist above left hand, face right wall. Weight is on right leg, right foot is turned out 45 degrees; left foot is on heel, knee extended, toes pointing up 45 degrees from floor.

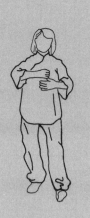

See front-view position of 11-H.

Checking the Whole Movement

■ Begin facing left wall; end facing right wall.

■ Begin with weight even; end with weight on right leg.

■ If right leg does not feel comfortable, bend it less.

■ If right knee does not feel comfortable, make sure that right foot is turned out 45 degrees.

■ If left leg does not feel hollow, move it closer to you.

■ If you do not feel balanced, be sure that your left leg is directly in front of your hip.

To end the movement, bring left heel to right heel and turn right foot parallel to left foot. Do the *Grand Movement*.

Repeat the sequence (11-F to 11-H), ending with the *Grand Movement*, four times or until you have the movements memorized. Shake your legs gently after each sequence. Then practice all of the movements you have learned, beginning with *Pay Respect to Mankind* and ending with the *Grand Movement*, twice. Shake your legs gently at the end of each sequence.

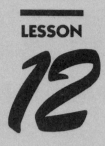

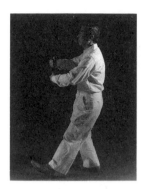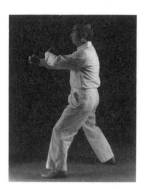

CARRY TIGER TO MOUNTAIN (SECOND HALF)

This movement is a pursuit of an opponent with your arms revolving in a circle to clear your way. It ends with delivering a punch to an opponent after your pursuit of him has been successful.

In this movement, as you lift your left foot, pay attention to inhalation. As you walk forward with your left foot and your hands circle clockwise left, pay attention to exhalation. When you walk forward with your right foot and your hands circle clockwise right, pay attention to inhalation. Use your intention to move your ch'i in a circle with your palms. If you keep your arms and legs relaxed, you should feel a wave of warm air circling around you as you walk. You take only two steps while making a full circle with your hands.

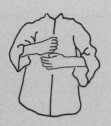

Arm Movement

12-A Place arms in the final position of *Carry Tiger to Mountain, First Half* (11-H).

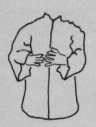

12-B Open right fist. Move left hand forward, palm facing right; right hand down, palm facing left. Keep elbows bent.

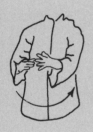

12-C Keeping hands in same relative position, circle arms from right to left, clockwise, forming the lower half of a small circle.

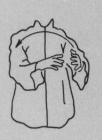

12-D Keeping hands in same relative position, circle arms from left to right, clockwise, forming the upper half of a small circle.

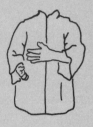

12-E With the upper half-circle almost complete and hands in front of you, make a loose fist with right hand and pull hand back to waist, knuckles down. Bring left hand closer to body, chest height, to form an arc with palm facing body.

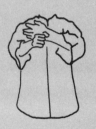

12-F Punch right hand forward under left hand, rotating fist 90 degrees to the left as you punch, keeping elbow slightly lowered. Move left forearm ahead as you punch, arms not touching.

Checking Yourself

- Hands circle clockwise: first right to left, then left to right.
- Punch slowly, right fist loose, rotating 90 degrees to left.
- Right fist and left forearm are moving forward as you punch.

Repeat the sequence of movements (12-A to 12-F) four times or until you have memorized it.

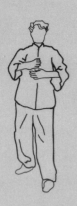

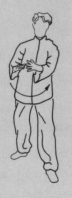

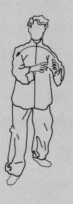

Leg Movement

12-G Stand in the final leg position of *Carry Tiger to Mountain, First Half* (11-H).

12-H Turn toe of left foot out 30 degrees and step down on foot. Shift weight to left leg, right leg hollow.

12-I Step forward on right foot, toe turned out 30 degrees. Shift weight to right leg, left leg hollow.

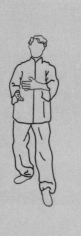

12-J Step forward on left foot, pointing toes ahead, bending knee forward slightly.

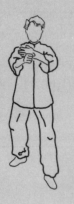

12-K Turn right foot out 60 degrees, bending knee out slightly. Sit in the middle in the *Two-Leg Solid Stance* (2-G), weight even.

Checking Yourself

- Face right wall.
- Pay attention to shifting your weight from left leg to right leg as you walk.
- If you do not feel comfortable at the end of the movement, make sure that your body is centered, your knees are bent evenly, right foot is turned out 60 degrees, and your left foot is directly in front of your hip.

Repeat the sequence of movements (12-G to 12-K) four times or until you have it memorized. Shake your legs gently at the end of each sequence.

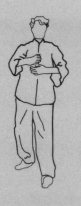

Combining Arm and Leg Movements

12-L Stand in the final position of *Carry Tiger to Mountain, First Half* (11-H), facing right wall.

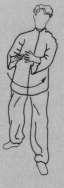

12-M Open right fist and move hands forward, left in front of right. Turn left foot out 30 degrees and step forward on it. Shift weight to left foot and move hands from right to left, forming a lower half-circle, without changing the relative position of each hand to the other.

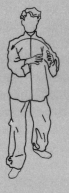

12-N Turn right foot out 30 degrees and step forward on it. Circle hands from left to right, forming an upper half-circle. Shift weight to right leg, left leg hollow.

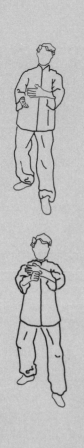

12-O Step forward on left foot, pointing toes ahead, bending knee forward slightly. Make a loose fist with right hand and pull hand back to waist, knuckles down. Form an arc with left forearm, chest height, palm in.

12-P Sit in the middle, weight even, and punch forward with right hand under left arm, rotating right fist to left 90 degrees as you punch. Pivot right toe out to 60 degrees.

Checking Yourself

- Face right wall.
- Walk slowly: first take a left step, then a right step.
- Shift weight fully: first to left leg, then to right leg.
- Make a small circle with your hands (6 to 8 inches) while you walk.
- Punch slowly, right fist loose, rotating fist to left.
- Check for comfort and balance.

To end the movement, bring right foot parallel to left foot, and do the *Grand Movement*.

Repeat the sequence (12-L to 12-P), ending with the *Grand Movement*, four times or until you have the sequence memorized. Then practice all the movements you have learned, from *Pay Respect to Mankind* to the *Grand Movement*, in a sequence twice. Shake your legs gently at the end of each sequence.

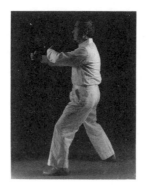 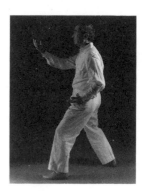

UNDER ELBOW BLOW

This movement symbolically suggests a downward deflection of an attacker's punch with the left hand and a facial blow to an opponent with the back of your right hand.

In this movement, your legs do not move. As you lower your right hand, pay attention to inhalation. At the same time, use your intention to bring your ch'i toward your body with your palm. As you extend your right hand forward and lower your left hand to your side, pay attention to exhalation. If you keep your arms and legs relaxed, you should feel a wave of warm air circling in front of your body.

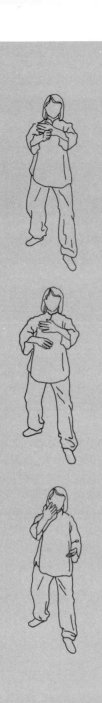

Combining Arm and Leg Movements

13-A Stand in the final position of *Carry Tiger to Mountain, Second Half* (12-P).

13-B Open right fist and pull right hand toward chest, elbow bent, palm in, arm parallel to floor.

13-C Bring left hand to left side, waist height, elbow bent, palm up. Strike forward with back of right hand.

Checking Yourself

- Strike with back of right hand.
- Right elbow partially bent.
- Left palm up, waist height, elbow bent.

Repeat the sequence of movements (13-A to 13-C) four times or until you have memorized it.

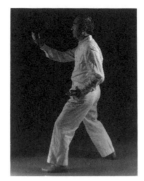
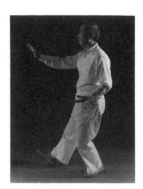

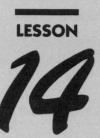

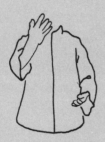

STEP BACK TO REPULSE MONKEY

This movement symbolically suggests the pulling of an attacker's arm with one hand and transferring his strength back to him with a push with the other hand while stepping backward.

In the beginning of this movement, as you pull with your right hand and shift your weight to the right leg, pay attention to inhalation. As you push with your left hand and make your left leg hollow, pay attention to exhalation. If your arms and legs are relaxed, you can feel your ch'i moving from the right arm to the left arm.

Arm Movement

14-A Place your arms in the final position of the *Under Elbow Blow* (13-C).

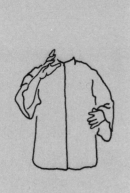

14-B Start to turn right palm down. Start to bring left palm up to chest level.

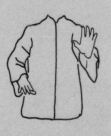

14-C Pull right arm down to waist, elbow bent, palm down. Push left arm forward, elbow slightly bent, palm forward.

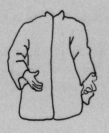

14-D Pull down left hand, turning left palm up. Turn right palm up, bringing up right hand.

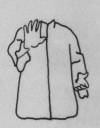

14-E Bring left hand to waist height, palm up. Push right hand forward at chest height, palm out.

Checking Yourself

- Begin: left arm pushing, right arm pulling (palm down).
- End: right arm pushing, left arm pulling (palm up).

Repeat the sequence of movements (14-A to 14-E) four times or until you have memorized it.

Now practice all of the movements you have learned, beginning with *Pay Respect to Mankind* and ending with the *Grand Movement*, twice. Shake your legs gently at the end of each sequence.

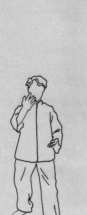

Leg Movement

14-F Stand in final leg position of *Under Elbow Blow* (13-C).

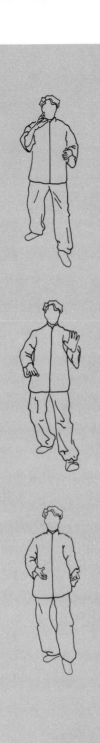

14-G Turn right foot in slightly (from 60 degrees to 45 degrees). Shift weight to right leg.

14-H Let left foot rest on heel, toe up, knee straight.

14-I Keeping weight on right foot, begin to step back with left foot.

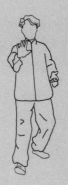

14-J Step back on left foot, keeping left leg on left side of body, turning toe out 45 degrees.

Checking Yourself

- If the bent leg does not feel comfortable, bend it less.
- If the straight leg does not feel hollow, move it closer to you.
- If you do not feel balanced, be sure that your straight leg is directly in front of your hip.

Repeat the sequence of movements (14-F to 14-J) four times or until you have it memorized. Shake your feet gently at the end of each sequence.

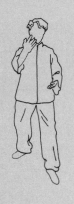

Combining Arm and Leg Movements

14-K Stand in the final position of the *Under Elbow Blow (13-C).*

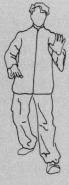

14-L Turn right foot in slightly (from 60 degrees to 45 degrees). Shift weight to right leg; bring left toe up. Pull right arm back, palm down, and bring left palm up. Push left palm forward.

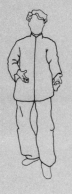

14-M Begin to step backward with left foot, keeping weight on right leg; turn left palm up and bring to waist. Turn right palm up.

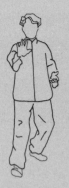

14-N Shift weight to left leg, turn toes out 45 degrees; keep right leg hollow, resting on heel, toes up. Push right arm forward, palm out.

Checking Yourself

■ Face right wall.
■ Check for comfort and balance. Keep torso erect and weight on left leg.

To end the movement, bring right foot parallel to left foot, and do the *Grand Movement*.

Repeat the whole movement, ending with the *Grand Movement*, in a sequence twice. Shake your legs gently at the end of each sequence.

LESSON

15

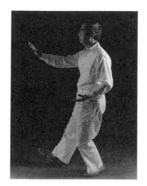 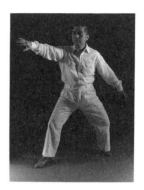

SLANTED PALMS FLYING AND THE T'AI CHI GRAND TERMINUS (THE GRAND MOVEMENT)

This movement symbolically suggests a retaliation after stopping an opponent's attack from below.

In this movement, when you turn your left foot and pull down with your open right hand, pay attention to inhalation. When you shift your weight to both legs and bring your arms up, pay attention to exhalation. At the same time, use your intention to move your ch'i with your arms. If you keep your arms and legs relaxed, you should feel a wave of warm air surrounding your body and extending from your arms to your legs.

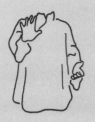

Arm Movement

15-A Place the arms in the final position of *Step Back to Repulse Monkey* (14-N).

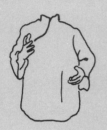

15-B Turn right palm to left as you start to bring right hand down toward abdomen. Move left palm toward abdomen.

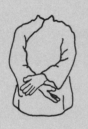

15-C Lower both hands to abdomen height: left hand in front of right, left palm in, right palm facing left and out. Hands and arms, crossing at wrists, do not touch each other or body; bend elbows slightly.

See close-up of hands in position 15-C.

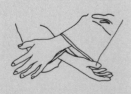

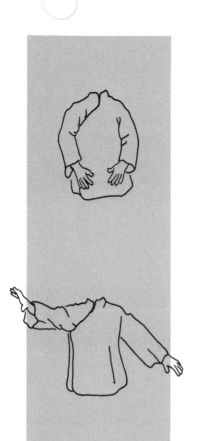

15-D Move hands apart in front of abdomen, turning right palm in. Right hand moves right, left hand moves left; palms in, fingers apart.

15-E Move right arm toward right corner; raise to shoulder height, elbow almost straight, palm back. Left arm moves toward left, to hip height, elbow almost straight, palm back.

Checking Yourself

- Arms in diagonal line, slightly curved, from right hand (high point) to left hand (low point).
- Elbows slightly bent.
- Palms face back.

Repeat the sequence of movements (15-A to 15-E) four times or until you have memorized it.

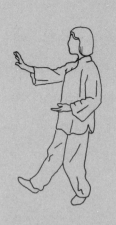

Leg Movement

15-F Stand in final leg position of *Step Back to Repulse Monkey* (14-N), facing right wall.

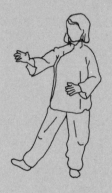

15-G Turn left to face front wall. Turn left foot out 45 degrees (toward left corner), pivoting on heel. Shift weight to left leg.

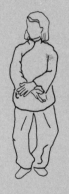

15-H Bring right heel to left heel, right leg hollow, left leg solid, toes pointing out 45 degrees (toward right corner).

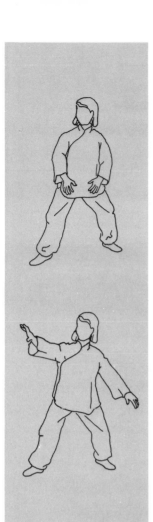

15-I With right foot, step toward right corner.

15-J Sit in the middle, weight even. Bend knees slightly.

Checking Yourself

- ■ Begin facing right wall; end facing front.
- ■ Shift from weight on left leg to weight evenly distributed on both legs.
- ■ End with right foot pointing toward right corner, left foot pointing toward left corner.

Repeat the sequence of movements (15-F to 15-J) four times or until you have it memorized. Shake your legs gently at the end of each sequence.

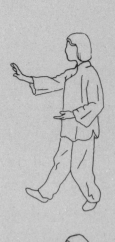

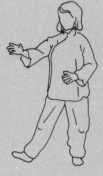

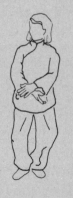

Combining Arm and Leg Movements

15-K Stand in the final position of *Step Back to Repulse Monkey* (14-N).

15-L Pivot on left foot to face front wall, weight on left leg, turning left foot out slightly, right leg hollow; pull right hand toward you and turn left palm in.

15-M Bring right heel to left heel: left leg solid, right leg hollow. Lower hands to height of abdomen, left wrist in front of right wrist. Right palm faces left and up; left palm faces in, hands not touching.

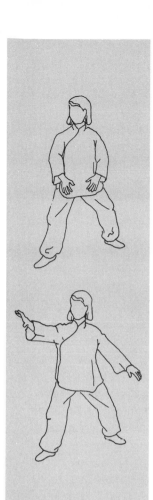

15-N With right foot, step toward right corner and move hands apart, palms in, right hand moving right, left hand moving left at the same pace.

15-O Sit in the middle with weight even, moving right arm toward right corner, a little above shoulder height, elbow almost straight, palm back. Move left arm toward back, elbow almost straight, palm back. Look toward right corner.

Checking Yourself

■ Body faces forward; face is turned toward right corner.
■ Arms are in a diagonal line from high (right hand) to low (left hand).

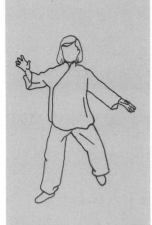

Now follow with the Grand Movement

15-P Transition: Starting from the final movement of *Slanted Palms Flying* (15-O), turn left foot 45 degrees to face front wall, shifting weight to left leg.

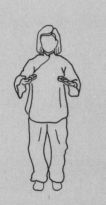

15-Q Bring right heel next to left heel and do the *Grand Movement*.

Repeat the sequence of *Slanted Palms Flying* and the *Grand Movement* four times or until you have it memorized. Shake your legs gently after each sequence.

Then practice all of the movements you have learned in a sequence twice. Shake your legs gently at the end of each sequence.

THE STANDING MEDITATION (THE UNIVERSAL POST)

This exercise, which strengthens the flow of vital energy throughout the body, can be done with the eyes open or closed. If you close your eyes, you can more easily feel the sensations of warmth that accompany the flow of energy.

Master Kuo recommended that students do the exercise after a set of T'ai Chi to round off each practice session with a moment of quiet. We also recommend it for relieving stress at the end of the day's work. Hold each position (right leg, left leg) from three to five minutes. As your legs and back become stronger, slowly increase the time.

In the beginning, your shoulders, arms, and legs will feel some strain after a few minutes of standing. Loosen them by shaking your arms and legs gently and shrugging your shoulders a few times. Shake your hands (and feet) as if you were shaking off drops of water.

Breathe slowly and naturally. As you stand, your breathing rate will decrease. Gradually, your breathing will be directed from your abdomen instead of your chest.

By calming the mind, relaxing the body, clearing your thoughts, and breathing naturally, you will become able to feel the flow of ch'i from your arms to your hands and to your feet. An early sign of the flow of ch'i is warmth on both your palms and the soles of your feet. You should not concentrate on these feelings; just let them happen naturally. Eventually, you will be able to feel your ch'i flow to every part of your body when you direct it with your intention.

After practicing this exercise and the sitting meditation for about a year, we could feel the effects of ch'i flow as a stream of warmth within the body, a stream that could be controlled by inhalation or exhalation. We felt a soothing sensation where ch'i passed through the body.

We further developed the power to control ch'i as we directed the ch'i flow while we performed individual movements of T'ai Chi. We practiced each movement slowly so that our body motion and breathing rhythm were synchronized with the flow of ch'i.

The Exercise

- To get ready: Facing front, stand with your feet together and parallel, holding your head erect but not stiff, as if a string were gently pulling up the top of your head.
- Let your shoulders drop.
- Let your weight "slide" down your arms to your hands and down your legs to your feet.
- Completely relax your abdomen.

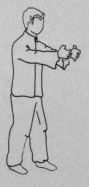

15-R Turn left foot to left corner (45 degrees) and shift weight to left leg. Move right leg slightly forward and let it rest lightly on the ball of the foot, toes pointed out 30 degrees. Extend arms and hands to form a circle in front of chest; keep elbows slightly bent at same level, palms in, fingertips overlapping but not touching, left hand closer to body. Leave a space of about two inches between the fingertips of your left and right hands.

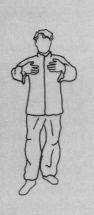

15-S See front view of exercise: weight on left foot, toes turned slightly toward left corner.

To Complete Exercise

■ Reverse your position, beginning again by checking posture—head erect, shoulders down. Let your body weight slide down to your feet, abdomen relaxed.

■ Turn right foot to right corner (45 degrees) and shift weight to right leg.

■ Move left leg slightly forward and rest it lightly on the ball of the foot, toes pointed out 30 degrees.

■ Extend arms and hands to form a circle in front of chest; keep elbows slightly bent at same level, right hand closer to body. Leave a space of about two inches between the fingertips of your left and right hands.

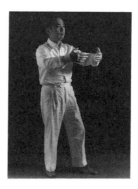

T'ai Chi Ch'uan / **151**

Think about muddy water:
If you try to stir the dirt out,
The more you stir
The muddier it gets.

How shall we have clear water?

Leave the muddy water alone.
The dirt will settle by itself.

In the same way we find contentment: Let each
  thing act according to its nature.
Give it time.
It will come to rest in its own way.

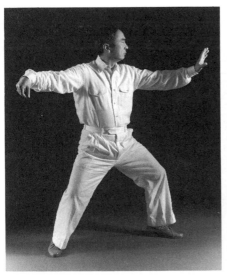
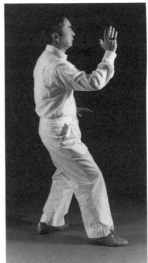
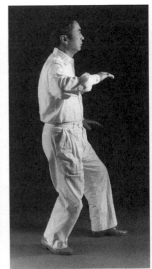

THE HEALING POWER OF T'AI CHI

Those who truly know the nature of existence
Push nothing to excess.
Because they do not push things to excess
They satisfy their needs again and again,
Yet exhaust nothing.

from Lao Tzu, *Tao Teh King*[1]

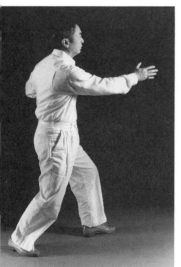 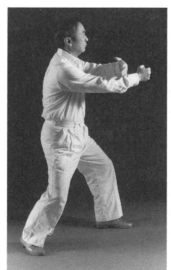 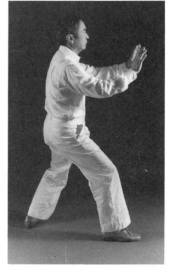

Now that you know how to practice Ch'i Kung and T'ai Chi, the aim of this chapter is simple: to show you, through the experience of others, what these healing arts can mean to you. Faithful practice is the key to the benefits of both, and faithful practice means daily practice. For long life, then, and health and happiness, practice daily.

PSYCHOSOMATIC DISORDERS

Many members of the healing professions are aware that millions of Americans suffer from psychosomatic disorders. Four to ten million people experience anxiety in the form of panic attacks, characterized by rapid, shallow breathing, an increased heart rate, and a sense of impending doom. As many doctors are also aware, severely anxious people experience biochemical responses that do not occur in normal people, for example, an oversensitivity to lactic acid, which the body produces during hard exercise, and to carbon dioxide, even in small quantities, such as in one's own breath.[2] Caffeine, too, in an amount equivalent to about four cups of coffee, can set off and magnify attacks of anxiety.[3] Many chemical changes observed in anxious people also occur among people suffering from another common disorder, depression, which, at any given time (because depression is a cyclical disorder), may afflict some 6 percent of the adult population.[4]

Together, these disorders trouble millions of Americans. Yet what can the healing professions tell us about these problems? Can they explain where anxiety and depression are located? Are they in the mind or in the body? Are they biochemical disorders or social and psychological problems? What should doctors prescribe for conditions like these? Psychoactive drugs like Valium and Elavil, or behavioral therapies like exposure to the feared situation and encouragement of a support group? And what of the side effects of drugs that doctors may prescribe?

Anxiety and depression are just two of many disorders that lie somewhere between body and mind. Some of the most painful physical conditions are psychosomatic. Allergies afflict millions of people every year, and arthritis brings discomfort, stiffness, and disabling pain to "some 15 million elderly Americans, at a cost exceeding $3.5 billion" in a typical year.[5] Yet no satisfactory treatment for these problems exists.

If our healing professions, with thousands of chemical substances at hand, cannot offer a known, consistently successful way of dealing with serious problems like these, why not try a different approach? To be sure, our approach is one that Western medicine cannot prove to be valid. But Western medicine has no proven approach of its own to offer. In circumstances like these, experience, filtered through long tradition, may be as good a guide as we are likely to find. As teachers of T'ai Chi know from self-observation and from students' reports, daily practice of T'ai Chi shows remarkable success in alleviating psychosomatic illnesses.

A PERSONAL SUCCESS STORY

My own story of regaining health is a T'ai Chi success story. Born in Canton, China, I joined my father in California when I was sixteen. For three years I worked in his market, where I was exposed to all sorts of allergens. I became accustomed to using up box after box of Kleenex. As a child I had suffered from asthma, and in California the illness returned.

My symptoms became more severe when I got a job in a laboratory where several people smoked cigars and pipes. After I had been there for a year my allergies were worse than ever. Finally, one day I had an attack of asthma so severe that an ambulance crew rushed me from the laboratory to the emergency room of the local hospital.

I learned about allergies for the first time during the days I spent at the hospital. Almost every pollen, mold, and house dust they scratched me with caused a reaction. For almost ten years I took allergy shots. Still my allergic condition came back each year from the end of February to the beginning of June.

One specialist who cared for me made me feel especially hopeless. Like the other doctors I had seen, he told me that allergy is a disease. But he was a fellow allergy sufferer. Seeing him with the same symptoms made me feel that nothing could cure this illness. Even so, because he knew about allergies from the inside, I decided to do everything he recommended except take allergy shots, which did not seem to work for me.

Following his advice, I used a disposable mask outdoors and an electronic air cleaner indoors during the allergy season. We gave away all woolen blankets and rugs and wiped the floor every day to keep down the dust. I watched my diet carefully and ate only the foods on the recommended list. Even with these precautions, I had hay fever and asthma for about four months each year.

THE TURNING POINT

My crisis became a turning point. As a teenager in China, I had studied martial arts. Now I determined to use them to rebuild my strength. Perhaps, I thought, if only I were stronger my condition would improve. During my teenage years I had outgrown my asthma. I now believed that "soft" martial arts practice was one reason why. As a teenager, besides studying several "hard" martial arts, I had learned T'ai Chi Ch'uan from a friend whose family had a teacher come to their home. My friend and I exchanged what we learned. We practiced martial arts as a sport—for fun, not for health.

Now I decided to learn T'ai Chi Ch'uan again. One day Emily saw a T'ai Chi Ch'uan studio not far from our home. The teacher was proud to show us photographs of his teacher, Kuo Lien-Ying. We decided to study with Master Kuo.

For the next five years, we rose every morning at 4:30 A.M., tucked our sleeping children into the car, and drove to San Francisco, where we met Master Kuo at his studio by 5:30 and practiced T'ai Chi at a park in front of his school. But it didn't happen just like that; first I had to persuade Master Kuo to take us as his private pupils.

MY FIRST T'AI CHI LESSON

Master Kuo was then in his early seventies, but he moved with the speed and grace of a twenty-year-old. More truly, he moved like a tiger. With his clean-shaven head, he reminded me of my martial arts teacher in Hong Kong, who had once been a Buddhist monk. But I could not tell the Master's age. He not only had the body of a young man; he looked at me with the piercing eyes of an eagle. When he spoke, his voice filled the studio.

"Why do you want to learn T'ai Chi Ch'uan?" he asked.

I told him I had been well-trained and a good student as a teenager and wanted to see what I remembered of my studies. "Do you want to see what I can do?" I asked.

"Don't bother," he replied. "Like everyone else you will have to start from the beginning."

I explained that I had to come fifty miles to San Francisco, and that I would not study with him unless he would teach me personally and privately. Master Kuo seemed to like my directness; he smiled and agreed.

When I met Master Kuo the next morning, I asked, "What is T'ai Chi?"

Master Kuo answered, "T'ai Chi is yin and yang working together."

I asked, "What are yin and yang?"

Master Kuo said, "Yin and yang are everything."

I responded, "Then T'ai Chi is everything working together as one thing."

He smiled.

I asked, "How do I learn T'ai Chi?"

Master Kuo replied, "By practicing T'ai Chi Ch'uan conscientiously." He paused for a moment and added, "You will know what T'ai Chi is when you can defeat an opponent who punches faster than you with no movement at all and when you can overcome his force of a thousand pounds with only eight ounces."

The following day, I found Master Kuo writing on the blackboard in the studio: "To move, let everything be moving together. To be still, let everything be still together."

That was our first lesson in the principle of T'ai Chi.

THE CHANGE COMES NATURALLY

We practiced conscientiously. Master Kuo's title of fourth-generation master had announced that he was a great master; his bearing made it clear. Though we began each day alone with Master Kuo, by 6:30 the park outside his studio would fill with students, all eager to learn from him or simply to practice near him.

Although, after practicing for a year, I did come down with asthma, the attack lasted only a couple of weeks, while the period for recovery was days instead of weeks. At the end of the season, having suffered about a quarter of the usual discomforts, I was very pleased with my progress. For the first time in many years, I did not miss a single day of work.

During my brief attack, I continued going to practice with Master Kuo. I wheezed, but at least I could breathe. Master Kuo, seeing I was having difficulty with the movements, taught me a standing T'ai Chi exercise that he called the "Universal Post." After a few days of practicing this movement, I was amazed to find that some of my hay fever symptoms disappeared. I then regularly practiced this exercise (see p. 149). As I later found out, the Universal Post is a Ch'i Kung exercise that Master Kuo had incorporated into his T'ai Chi training.

As I conscientiously practiced, week by week I grew stronger and grew well. Some will say I got over my allergies because I believed I would. Master Kuo would say I had learned to work with the yin and yang elements and to develop internal healing power. However it came about, after two years of T'ai Chi Ch'uan, fifteen years of allergies were gone.

MANY STORIES OF SUCCESS

Stories of healing through T'ai Chi are familiar to everyone who practices it. Among our students, we have seen astonishing improvements. Several students have taken up T'ai Chi after finding no relief from arthritis. One student, a furniture refinisher, had been diagnosed as having a degenerative arthritic condition affecting his shoulders, hands, and upper arms. He found that with T'ai Chi his pain disappeared. As with my allergies, the improvement began remarkably soon. He writes:

> I could not sleep on either side for two years—only flat on my back. I had to take aspirin three times each night to be able to sleep. I had extreme pain putting on my undershirt as well as extending my left arm above my head.
>
> Within the third and fourth month of T'ai Chi lessons, my arthritis pain had reduced to the point that I no longer required taking aspirin and began enjoying sleeping on both left and right sides. My pain disappeared. I regained full use of my left arm and was able to extend it in any direction without pain. Within six to eight months, I was totally free from any effects of arthritis.[6]

According to this student's wife, he had been suffering pain for nearly seven years. He had given up taking drugs after a few years because of their side effects. Yet he began to regain his flexibility, his energy, and his sense of well-being after only six weeks of practicing T'ai Chi.

Another student, an older woman whose hands were badly swollen by arthritis, reported,

> I find that my hands are now mobile to the point of closing into a fist—and the swelling has diminished to such an extent that I cannot wear my rings without losing them because the rings had been enlarged to fit the arthritic hand.[7]

Another found that practicing T'ai Chi and Ch'i Kung helped both arthritis and back pain:

> About two years ago I began to develop a stiffness and pain in my hands. My fingers were so stiff, swollen, and sore that I had difficulty holding a toothbrush. My hands did not have the strength to lift ordinary objects like a half-gallon carton of milk. I could not turn the knobs on the shower with one hand. Upon medical examination, it was determined there was not much I could do but live with it and keep exercising while taking aspirin for the pain. Altogether it was a very frightening and discouraging experience.
>
> My wife and I began taking your T'ai Chi class and things began to happen. After the first two or three months, my hands and fingers began working better. Movement came back and pain subsided. By mid-January the arthritis symptoms had almost disappeared. My wedding ring and another ring I had worn for years slipped onto my fingers again, after I had not been able to wear them for over a year and a half. Today, my hands and fingers are perfectly normal.
>
> At the same time, I have had a lower back condition for over twenty-five years and have had my back "go out" on me from time to time. I have made regular visits to the chiropractor during all that time for adjustments and general maintenance. Generally, upon standing on two scales, one foot on each, in the chiropractor's office, my weight has been about 15 pounds heavier on one side owing to the imbalance in my lower back. Today the difference is about 2 pounds, which is perfectly normal. Again, T'ai Chi and Ch'i Kung have come to the rescue.
>
> Both my wife and I feel better, have more energy, and generally feel "up" all the time. Both of us have always been very positive

thinkers (as you know, I am a Dale Carnegie instructor), but that positiveness is constantly being reinforced within us through our practice of T'ai Chi and Ch'i Kung.[8]

This student found his hands so fully restored to mobility that he bought a new piano.

A study of arthritic patients at the University of Illinois College of Medicine shows that the experience of our students occurs in other settings as well:

> After ten weeks of practicing T'ai Chi Ch'uan, seven people decreased the time it took to walk 50 feet by 17.7 percent; their grip strength increased 32.6 percent in the right arm and 40.7 percent in the left, and the amount of joint tenderness dropped 37.5 percent.[9]

Migraine headaches, too, respond to T'ai Chi. One of our students, a technical editor for Apple Computer, has described her experience:

> For almost twenty years before learning T'ai Chi, I got severe migraine headaches, usually once or twice a month. These were the classic migraines, complete with blurred vision and nausea. I'd be bedridden for an entire day, and would still feel some pain the day after. Various types of medication were prescribed but didn't help. Since learning T'ai Chi in 1976, however, I've had only a few migraines; these happened at times of unusually high stress but were minor and didn't last long. There's no doubt that this improvement is due to the beneficial effects of T'ai Chi on my mind and body.[10]

T'AI CHI AND THE OFFICE

Though the practice of T'ai Chi can have a positive effect on psycho-somatic illnesses, it offers an even greater benefit. By helping to prevent a build-up of stress, T'ai Chi helps healthy people stay well and strong. To illustrate, consider the experience of another student, who had learned many lessons of T'ai Chi: how to relax, to breathe smoothly, and to control his inner energy with his thoughts. He found that these skills became survival skills at work:

> My phone rang, and the person calling told me there was a serious

problem with some work I had just finished. He said it looked like a big error and he would call me back soon to let me know just how badly I had messed things up. He sounded angry.

When I hung up the phone I just sat there and thought about breathing. After I had taken three or four long deep breaths, my mind was calm. If I had made an error, I was ready to fix it. If someone was angry with me, I could wait until he cooled down.

Just as I was thinking to myself, "Two years ago I'd have been climbing the wall over this," the phone rang again. It was the person who had just called me. "Sorry," he said. "The mistake was ours. Your work is fine."[11]

Stressful moments like these overtake us every day. You don't need an opponent rushing at you to find yourself in physical danger; your own response to stress can raise your blood pressure, speed up your heartbeat, and cause you to breathe in an irregular way. The impulse toward "fight or flight" still works in us as it did in our distant ancestors.

Many people prepare for stress by building up the muscles of heart and lungs through vigorous cardiovascular exercise like racquetball or jogging. There is, however, another way: you can also take care of your heart by teaching body and mind to cushion it from shocks and by strengthening it from within, using ch'i. Emotional stress is like a violent enemy that attacks us from within. Fortunately, by practicing the lessons of T'ai Chi Ch'uan you can learn to deflect it. A calm mind, relaxation, regular breathing, and controlled movement can turn aside an "inside" attack of stressful emotions. To paraphrase the ancient adage, with T'ai Chi Ch'uan you can "turn aside a force of a thousand pounds *of emotion* with just eight ounces *of intention*." T'ai Chi Ch'uan trains us to sidestep stress and deal calmly with problems *as* problems. T'ai Chi not only heals our bodies, it helps us practice the prevention that is better than any cure.

HEALING

Healing of the body is a natural process. Everyone has seen it work hundreds of times and with all kinds of injuries—from a mosquito bite to a hole left by a baby tooth to deep cuts and badly broken bones. In China, acupuncture and acupressure are considered ways of facilitating this natural healing process. It is not surprising, then, to find that many illnesses Chinese doctors treat by acupuncture respond to the practice of T'ai Chi Ch'uan. As the Chinese doctors explain, the flow of internal energy or ch'i promotes healing. When that flow is weak or intermittent, the body cannot fully or rapidly recover from the many large and small injuries it receives during the course of ordinary living. When the flow is strong and regular, the power of ch'i can heal nerves, muscles, and membranes, so that illnesses like allergies, headaches, high blood pressure, back pain, and arthritis disappear. When your body is relaxed, your mind calm, and your breathing and movements smooth and balanced, the body will heal itself naturally.

REPLENISH YOURSELF

A lesson from a child gave me insight into a way of thinking that can help us all. Emily and I had gone to back-to-school night. Our daughter's third-grade teacher welcomed the parents by sharing with us an assignment she had given as a way of finding out more about each child in the class. She had asked each child to make a list of twenty-five things he or she did well. Our daughter's list began, "Helping my mother." It ended, "Loving myself."

Helping others and loving yourself go together. All of us spend time doing things for others. Most of us go to work. Most of us care for a family, household, or friends. With schedules and responsibilities uppermost in our minds, we often save little time to replenish our own energy and our inner selves. T'ai Chi can do that for us. The exercises you have learned give you fifteen minutes of tranquil movement each day. These exercises will prepare you to meet each day with strength and calmness or to relax and free yourself from stress after the day's work.

After work, or during the day, you may need a few minutes just for yourself. Six or seven minutes of sitting meditation or standing T'ai Chi meditation (*the Universal Post*) will calm you and relieve the day's tension.

With these practices and your daily sequence of T'ai Chi, you will strengthen your inner power, your vital energy. What better way to seek health, happiness, and well-being than this? Those who learn how to care for themselves by faithfully practicing T'ai Chi find inner strength and vitality they never dreamed they might possess. They have learned the truth of the old philosopher's words:

> Those who truly know the nature of existence
> Push nothing to excess.
> Because they do not push things to excess
> They satisfy their needs again and again,
> Yet exhaust nothing.

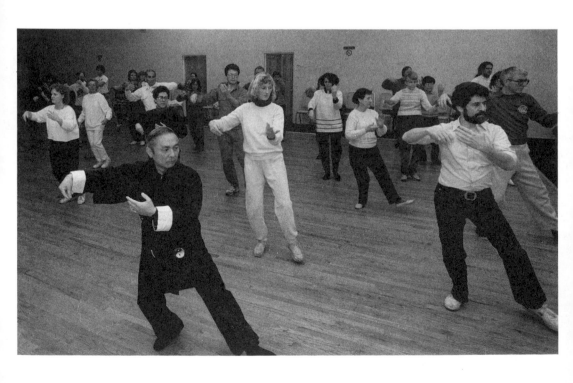

OPTIMIZING YOUR FITNESS SYSTEM

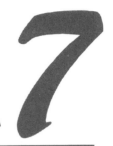

The human being, like the whole of nature, is a *system*. Inner observation, the study of T'ai Chi, and my engineer's habit of orderly analysis have led me to break up this system into four parts: the body, the mind, the flow of energy in the body, and the flow of thoughts in the mind. If part of the system functions poorly, the whole system will be impaired. The crucial thing is to keep the flow of energy going smoothly throughout the body and the flow of thought going smoothly throughout the mind. This is, you might say, an electrical engineer's view of how we work. But when you work, as I do, with systems like accelerators and computers, systems that depend upon electrical power, you see how important is the principle of flow. For the greatest flow of power— enough to turn on all the lights in San Francisco—can be blocked by the smallest imperfection in the system. A tiny connector fails to connect, and the enterprise comes to a standstill.

The human system is even more complex than our computers and accelerators. Is it not logical to think that in it, too, some tiny "glitch" can cause trouble in the whole? Or, conversely, that keeping the current running can help the system reestablish its balance? If this is so, then a system of movement designed to promote the flow of energy and the flow of consciously directed thought might well have a positive effect on health. As we know from experience, T'ai Chi, this practical set of exercises refined by many generations of teachers and students, does have a powerful positive effect.

OPTIMAL WELLNESS

To me, the yin-yang circle stands for youth and well-being. At the same time it tells us in a symbolic way how to preserve these qualities.

The two halves of the circle represent the self and wellness (or robust health), two interdependent parts of one whole. How many times have you heard someone say, "I'm so tired that I'm not myself today"? When the self is impaired, whether by fatigue or illness or emotional turbulence, it seems to lose its nature. When the self and wellness are united, we feel whole and complete. We are one: strong as the perfect form, a circle; and full, like a circle, with a sense of well-being. The philosopher Lao Tzu praised oneness and connected it with the serenity of a clear sky, the solidity of undisturbed earth, and the fertility of unimpaired nature:

> Heaven in virtue of the One is limpid;
> Earth in virtue of the One is settled;
> The valley in virtue of the One is full;
> It is the One that makes these what they are.[1]

To carry this interpretation a step further, the self controls wellness as wellness affects the self. If we take wellness as the dark side of the yin-yang circle, we see that it contains a small circle of light. This symbolizes the power of the self—of attitude, mind, or thought—over our well-being.

TOP DOWN OR BOTTOM UP?

The T'ai Chi circle is a powerful and universal symbol. Less universal, but a powerful and personal symbol to me, is the computer. At a basic physical level, a computer is a set of on/off switches. The language the computer speaks, machine language, is a binary language composed of two words: "switch on" and "switch off." Yet a computer can control the processes that run an automobile assembly plant, a steel mill, or an accelerator for high-energy physics research. Or it can call upon vast stores of data and print out, in language humans can understand, the diagnosis of a disease, the outcome of a set of equations, or the titles of fifty recent articles on stress.

What links this physical machine with its yes-no language to the high-level abstractions of atomic physics? It is a computer program, a series of definitions and instructions that tell a computer how to perform a task. At the high end, a program is linked to an abstraction—the complex aim in the mind of a user. At the low end, it translates into machine code—the language of on and off. How to break down abstractions into instructions appropriate to the architecture of a machine or how to build complex abstractions using a machine's limited language—this is the job of the programmer.

Programming can be done either "bottom up" or "top down." Bottom-up programming begins with a machine, its character and limitations. In this method, "the lowest levels of instructions are combined to form a higher level operation which in turn may be used in the formulation of even higher level routines."[2] Bottom-up programming begins with the details. Top-down programming, on the other hand, begins with a simple overall structure. It then breaks this structure down into smaller components, describing and refining these at each level until a whole structure is fully detailed.

My work is top-down control of accelerators. I begin with what a team at SLAC wants an accelerator to do, translate this intention into mathematical equations, and see that these become a computer-based model of the accelerator's performance. If all goes well, a beam of particles strikes where and how it should, and a step in an experiment is carried through. If something goes wrong, I study the problem from both ends. If something has gone wrong with the accelerator's machinery, or the computer's hardware, or the details of the program, the problem must be solved bottom up. But often, the solution to the problem is found at the top. It is the intention or its expression in equations and model that need to be changed.

For me, this process is an apt metaphor for the self-guided practice of T'ai Chi: the mind forms an intention, the thoughts (like equations) create a model of this intention, the ch'i (like electrical signals) follows the model and guides the body, and the body responds. T'ai Chi is a top-down process. This process is full of power: it not only controls your physical movements, making them smoother, better coordinated, and more relaxed, but also strengthens your self. Controlling the movements of your body strengthens your control over mind and will. This is why students of T'ai Chi find themselves better able to achieve their goals.

But the T'ai Chi movements also work from the bottom up: as the body moves it stirs up the ch'i. The regular flow of ch'i improves the performance of the body and at the same time orders the thoughts. Thus from the top down or the bottom up, the slow, regular, ordered movements of T'ai Chi join the body and mind together into unity. Practicing T'ai Chi Ch'uan forms a feedback system that by closely coupling mind and body improves the performance and quality of both.

OPTIMIZING THE WHOLE SYSTEM

To use another metaphor, practicing T'ai Chi activates what I call the "fitness system." (See Figure 7-1.) Learning to control mind and body through thoughts and ch'i means practicing action and controlling action. This control means that we can act on others to enhance the harmony between ourselves and them. The results? *Harmony:* getting along easily with others. *Health:* equilibrium and wholeness of mind and body. *Healing:* the process by which the body repairs the damage of ordinary wear and tear. *Happiness:* the good feeling you have when both your mind and body are untroubled.

These four attributes—the power of self-healing, the equilibrium of health, happiness within ourselves, and harmony with those around us—are essential to the self. They form a system; if one fails, the others fail, too. If we drew them in a diagram (as in Figure 1-2, page 14), they would be the four sides of a square, each essential to the others. If we cannot get along with others, we lose our happiness. Loss of happiness affects, through the mind, the healing processes that maintain the body's health. Conversely, an injury that does not heal or an illness that lingers diminishes our happiness and our ability to get along with others.

Figure 7-1
This figure illustrates the T'ai Chi fitness system. T'ai Chi exercises mind and body, thoughts and ch'i. Through T'ai Chi you practice mental and physical action, internal and external exercise. By strengthening from the inside your control over your actions, you prepare yourself to gain harmony (getting along with others), health (caring for yourself), healing (letting nature do its work without hindrance), and happiness (the result of all the rest).

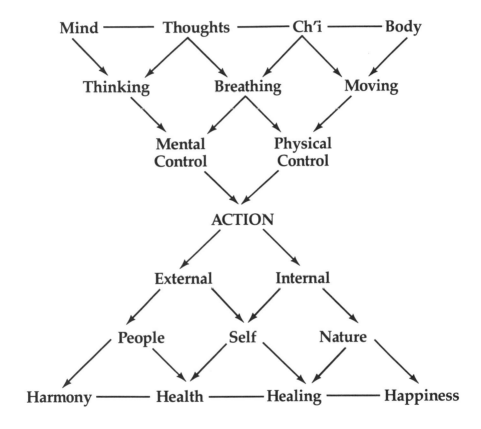

When the gentle, rhythmic movements of T'ai Chi have a healing effect on some illnesses and injuries, or when the calming effect of these same movements enhances harmony and happiness, T'ai Chi, by working on one of these processes, works on all. By benefiting the whole fitness system, it helps us all to achieve optimal well-being.

NOTES

Chapter 1

1. These personal statements come from students in the classes of 1985 to 1988.

Chapter 2

1. *Tao Teh King* by Lao Tzu, *Interpreted as Nature and Intelligence* by Archie J. Bahm (New York: Frederick Ungar Publishing, 1958), p. 60.
2. Quoted in Fritjof Capra, *The Turning Point: Science, Society, and the Rising Culture* (New York: Bantam Books, 1983), p. 62.
3. Deng Ming-Dao, *The Wandering Taoist* (San Francisco: Harper & Row, 1983), pp. 115–16.
4. Capra, *The Turning Point*, p. 314.
5. David Eisenberg, *Encounters with Qi* (New York: Penguin Books, 1987), pp. 89–90.
6. Ibid., p. 43.
7. Ibid., p. 44.
8. *The New York Times* (2 December 1986): p. 18.
9. Capra, *The Turning Point*, p. 314.
10. Michael Browning (Knight-Ridder News Service), "Take 220 Volts and Call Me Later," *The San Jose Mercury News* (7 January 1988).
11. "Electricity Promising in Treating Ulcers," *The San Jose Mercury News* (25 June 1987).
12. Shiao-Lin is the name of a famous Buddhist temple in northwest China, where, as recently as a hundred years ago, 3000 monks studied Buddhism and martial arts. (A popular television show tells the fictional adventures of a Shiao-Lin monk in California.)
13. At San Jose State University with William Winter, a professor of psychology, and in Palo Alto with Benjamin Chen, a physics professor from the University of California at Riverside.
14. The experiment, by physicians at Western Reserve University, is described by Edward Maisel in *Tai Chi for Health* (New York: Holt, Rinehart and Winston, 1972), pp. 53–54. (First published in 1963.)

15. Gordon Rattray Taylor, *The Natural History of the Mind* (New York: Penguin, 1981), pp. 145–46.
16. *The New York Times* (2 December 1986).

Chapter 3

1. Lao Tzu, *Tao Teh King, Interpreted as Nature and Intelligence*, translated by Archie J. Bahm, p. 12 (adapted by JoAn Johnstone).
2. Wang Tsung-Yueh was said to be the foremost pupil of Chang San-Feng, the traditional source of Tai Chi Ch'uan. He is the assigned author of a commentary on an earlier text on T'ai Chi. This translation is taken from Kuo Lien-Ying, *Tai Chi Chuan in Theory and Practice* (n. p. [Taiwan], n. d.), 7. The translator is anonymous.
3. Eisenberg, *Encounters with Qi*, p. 37.
4. Kuo Lien-Ying, *Tai Chi Chuan*, p. 3.
5. "How Brain Programs Itself to Concentrate on Tasks," *The San Jose Mercury News* (3 February 1987).
6. In the experiment Gevins directed, seven men were fitted with electrodes on their scalps and asked to respond quickly to a number flashed on a video screen. They pressed a button corresponding to the number they saw (Nos. 1 through 9 were used), while electrodes recorded changes in voltage from the group of neurons near each electrode. The researchers compared the shape of the waves recorded by different pairs of electrodes. Similar wave shapes, they concluded, meant that those areas of the brain were performing related functions. Next they mapped similar signals. They found that just before the men pushed the buttons, different groups of neurons near the surface of their brains began to interact with each other. Activity in the networks began as the men concentrated on the task, getting ready to respond. Even more interesting, the maps for answers that turned out to be right were frequently different from maps of incorrect answers. Two-thirds of the time, by examining the paths of connection set up by the brain in the split second before the men moved to press the button, researchers could predict whether the forthcoming answers would be correct or incorrect.
7. Taylor, *The Natural History of the Mind*, pp. 62–63.
8. Chang San-Feng, in Kuo, *Tai Chi Chuan*, p. 1.
9. [Wu Yu-Hsiang], in Kuo, *Tai Chi Chuan*, p. 3.
10. Personal letter, 1987.
11. Chang San-Feng, trans. by Benjamin Pang Jeng Lo, *The Essence of T'ai Chi Ch'uan*, (Berkeley, Calif.: North Atlantic Books, 1979), p. 22.
12. Personal letter, 1987.
13. Lao Tzu, *Tao Teh King* (adapted by JoAn Johnstone).
14. Emmett E. Miller with Deborah Lueth, *Self Imagery: Creating Your Own Good Health* (Berkeley, Calif.: Celestial Arts, 1986), p. 52. (Updated edition; first edition published by Prentice Hall, 1978.)
15. Lao Tzu, *Tao Teh King*, p. 66 (adapted by JoAn Johnstone).
16. Wang Tsung-Yue in *Tai Chi Chuan* by Kuo Lien-Ying.
17. Lawrence Galante, *Tai Chi the Supreme Ultimate* (York Beach, Maine: Samuel Weiser, 1981), pp. 23–25. The author mistakenly gives Wang's name as Wong and his age as 114.
18. Eisenberg, *Encounters with Qi*, pp. 40–41.
19. "Man Takes 115-Foot Fall to Dodge Car," *The San Jose Mercury News* (22 January 1988).

Chapter 4

1. David Eisenberg, *Encounters with Qi* (New York: Viking Penguin, 1987), pp. 139, 146–47, 224–25.
2. Joseph Needham, quoted in Edward Maisel, *Tai Chi for Health* (New York: Holt, Rinehart, and Winston, 1972), pp. 28–29.

Chapter 5

1. Photograph in Lawrence Galante, *Tai Chi: The Supreme Ultimate* (York Beach, Maine: Samuel Weiser, 1981), p. 18.
2. Illustration in Mark Salzman, "Wushu: Meditation in Motion," *The New York Times Magazine*, Part 2, 29 March 1987.
3. In the translation by Benjamin Pang Jeng Lo, *The Essence of T'ai Chi Ch'uan* (Berkeley, CA: North Atlantic Books, 1979).

Chapter 6

1. Lao Tzu, *Tao Teh King* (adapted by JoAn Johnstone).
2. Scott M. Fishman and David V. Sheehan, "Anxiety and Panic: Their Cause and Treatment," *Psychology Today* (April 1985), pp. 26–30.
3. M.P. Shanahan and R.N. Hughes, "Potentiation of Performance-Induced Anxiety by Caffeine in Coffee," *Psychological Reports* 59 (August 1986), pp. 83–86.
4. "Depression," *Newsweek* (4 May 1987), p. 48.
5. Joseph A. Califano, Jr., "The Health-Care Chaos," *The New York Times Magazine* (March 20, 1988), p. 58. The year for which the figures are given is 1987.
6. Personal letter, March 6, 1984.
7. Personal letter, February 10, 1984.
8. Personal letter, November 15, 1982.
9. Reported in *Weekly World News* (26 August 1986), p. 5.
10. Personal letter, October 1987.
11. Personal anecdote, April 1987.

Chapter 7

1. Lao-tzu, *Tao Teh Ching*, trans. by D. C. Lau (Baltimore: Penguin Books, 1963), p. 100 (adapted by JoAn Johnstone).
2. Dennis Longley and Michael Shain, *Dictionary of Information Technology* (New York: Oxford University Press, 1986), p. 38.

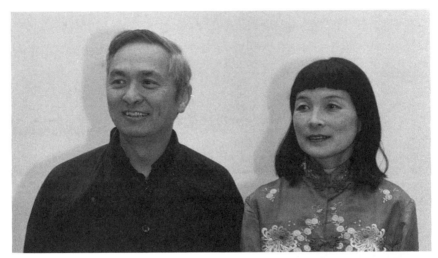

Martin and Emily Lee

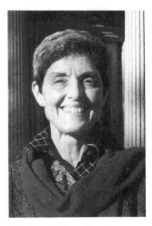

JoAn Johnstone

ABOUT THE AUTHORS

Emily Lee

Born in China, Emily Lee moved to Taiwan when she was 10 and then to the United States when she was 17. She and Martin Lee met and married when they were undergraduates at the University of California at Berkeley.

Mrs. Lee began her martial arts training in 1968. Soon after her studies began, she knew that she had found the subject she really wanted to master—the philosophy and practice of Chinese internal martial arts. During her ten years of study with Master Kuo Lien-Yin, founder of the Lien-Yin T'ai Chi Chuan School in San Francisco, she mastered both T'ai Chi Chuan and Pa Kua Chuan, an internal martial art that requires great physical and mental discipline. Emily Lee was the only woman whom Master Kuo accepted as a student of his most treasured art, Pa Kua Chuan.

After five years of intensive training, with the permission of her teacher, Emily began teaching T'ai Chi Chuan with her husband—a tremendously valuable community contribution they have continued for twenty years. Together they founded the T'ai Chi Cultural Center in 1978.

As a result of her understanding of the principles and philosophy behind Hsing Yi and Ch'i Kung—the result of two years of full-time study with Professor Yu Pen-Shi and his wife, Ou-Yang Min, who were her live-in masters—Mrs. Lee became one of the most popular and inspirational teachers in the Bay Area. She is one of the few women T'ai Chi masters who is expert in the complete system of the Chinese martial arts.

Martin Lee

Born and raised in China, Martin Lee came as a teenager to Stockton, California, where he attended the last two years of high school and junior college. He earned his B.S. from the University of California at Berkeley in 1960, his M.S from New York University in 1962, and his Ph.D. from Stanford University in 1967—all in electrical engineering.

Dr. Lee's career has encompassed two years (1960–1962) as a staff member at the Bell Telephone Laboratory, five years (1962–1967) as a microwave engineer at the Stanford Linear Accelerator Center (SLAC), and two years (1967–1969) as an accelerator physicist at the Brookhaven National Laboratory. Since 1969 he has been an engineering physicist at SLAC.

Now an internationally recognized expert in the field of accelerator control systems, Dr. Lee has published more than fifty technical papers and has served as consultant to accelerator centers and laboratories worldwide, as well as to many of the aerospace companies and defense industries in the United States.

As he recounts in his introduction, Dr. Lee found in T'ai Chi the cure for his severe allergies and asthma, and his studies led to his present status as T'ai Chi master. Thanks to his scientific training and interest, Dr. Lee was able to develop a systematic approach to the understanding and practice of T'ai Chi and Ch'i Kung. He and his wife, Emily, have instituted a course on T'ai Chi for total fitness in which they have taught thousands of students. They have also produced a videotape, MIND-BODY FITNESS, as a visual complement to this guide to the path to health via T'ai Chi.

JoAn Johnstone

JoAn Johnstone was born in Corvallis, Oregon. She attended Pomona College in Claremont, California, and earned a doctorate in English literature at the University of California in Berkeley. She has taught English at Stanford University, Hunter College, and several California community colleges. For a number of years she has worked as an editor associated with editcetera, a freelancers' group in Berkeley. She now lives in Middletown, Connecticut, with her husband, William Chace, president of Wesleyan University. She teaches an introductory class in T'ai Chi at Wesleyan.

CREDITS